Retroperitoneal Trauma

edited by

Scott B. Frame, M.D., F.A.C.S.
Assistant Professor
Division of Trauma/Critical Care
Department of Surgery
University of Tennessee
Graduate School of Medicine
Knoxville, Tennessee

Norman E. McSwain, Jr., M.D., F.A.C.S.
Professor
Department of Surgery
Tulane University School of Medicine
New Orleans, Louisiana

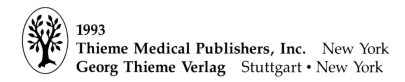
1993
Thieme Medical Publishers, Inc.   New York
Georg Thieme Verlag   Stuttgart • New York

Thieme Medical Publishers, Inc.
381 Park Avenue South
New York, New York 10016

RETROPERITONEAL TRAUMA
Scott B. Frame
Norman E. McSwain

Library of Congress Cataloging-in-Publication Data

Retroperitoneal Trauma / edited by Scott B. Frame, Norman E. McSwain, Jr.

    p.   cm.
    Includes bibliographical references and index.
    ISBN 0-86577-360-2 (Thieme Medical Publishers). -- ISBN
3-13-792301-8 (Georg Thieme Verlag)
    1. Retroperitoneum--Wounds and injuries. 2. Retroperitoneum-
-Surgery. I. Frame, Scott B. II. McSwain, Norman E., 1937-
    [DNLM: 1. Retroperitoneal Space--injuries. WI 575 R4378]
RD540.R48 1992
617.5'5044--dc20
DNLM/DLC   92-49416
for Library of Congress   CIP

Important note: Medicine is an ever-changing science. Research and clinical experience are continually broadening our knowledge, in particular our knowledge of proper treatment and drug therapy. Insofar as this book mentions any dosage or applications, readers may rest assured that the authors, editors, and publishers have made every effort to ensure that such references are strictly in accordance with the state of knowledge at the time of production of the book. Nevertheless, every user is requested to carefully examine the manufacturers' leaflets accompanying each drug to check on his own responsibility whether the dosage schedules recommended therein or the contraindications stated by the manufacturers differ from the statements made in the present book. Such examination is particularly important with drugs that are either rarely used or have been newly released on the market.

Some of the product names, patents, and registered designs referred to in this book are in fact registered trademarks or proprietary names even though specific reference to this fact is not always made in the text. Therefore, the appearance of a name without designation as proprietary is not to be construed as a representation by the publisher that it is in the public domain.

Printed in the United States of America.

5   4   3   2   1

TMP ISBN 0-86577-360-2
GTV ISBN 3-13-792301-8

Contents

Preface

The abdomen in trauma has often been likened to a "black box" in which injuries may occur. These injuries are a frequent cause of preventable trauma deaths in most large series such as the Orange and Dade County studies. Much attention has been given to diagnosing intra-abdominal injuries, and diagnostic peritoneal lavage has revolutionized the ability to diagnose these injuries. However, the retroperitoneum has remained a source of missed injuries and etiology of both early and late morbidity and mortality in the trauma patient. The retroperitoneal structures are separated from the intra-abdominal cavity by the posterior peritoneum. This peritoneal barrier renders diagnostic peritoneal lavage highly inaccurate for the diagnosis of injuries in the retroperitoneum. This region, therefore, represents a distinct entity in trauma care which presents very difficult problems to the physician caring for the trauma patient. Injuries to the major vascular structures may cause very early mortality if not recognized and treated, and can present therapeutic challenges to the surgeon when confronted with these difficult-to-expose injuries. Missed injuries in the retroperitoneum challenge the physician as diagnostician. Mortality from retroperitoneal hematomas averages around 20%, and this rate has not changed in the past 20 years.

This book will address the retroperitoneum as a separate and distinct entity in the care of the trauma patient. A thorough understanding of retroperitoneal anatomy is essential to fully appreciate the injuries that may occur and the diagnostic and operative techniques that must be employed to identify and treat these difficult injuries. The manner in which a patient is initially evaluated will be reviewed, and special techniques and studies necessary to identify retroperitoneal injuries will be covered. For the clinician to have a complete understanding of retroperitoneal injuries and maintain the proper index of suspicion for their presence, an understanding of the mechanisms of injury which result in retro-peritoneal injuries is essential. The kinematics of retroperitoneal injuries is therefore discussed. Retroperitoneal hematomas remain a challenge to the operating surgeon when he is confronted with one at the time of surgical exploration. The trauma surgeon must have a systematic approach to abdominal exploration and the management of retroperitoneal hematomas when they are found. Sound surgical technique for proper exposure of injuries is essential and is discussed in detail. Computed tomography has exploded on the medical and trauma scene as a means of evaluating the trauma patient and has become a valuable tool in diagnosing retroperitoneal injuries. This is discussed thoroughly by two of the major experts in the field of CT scanning in abdominal trauma. Finally, each organ system in the retroperitoneum is discussed individually, with special diagnostic techniques presented, which are peculiar for that organ system, and proper surgical management of injuries are reviewed.

It is hoped that this book will serve as a valuable reference tool for all physicians caring for the trauma patient. Much of the book is devoted to specific organ injury management, which will obviously be of value to the general surgeon confronted with trauma patients. It is also hoped that this text will be of benefit to all emergency physicians and others who are responsible for the early care of trauma patients so that proper initial evaluation and diagnostic procedures will be carried out for the early diagnosis of injuries in the retroperitoneum.

The contributors to this monograph all have extensive experience in the care of trauma patients in the respective fields in which they are writing. Many are recognized national and international leaders in their respective fields and bring to this monograph the benefit of their extensive knowledge, research, and experience in the care of trauma patients. Grateful acknowledgment must also be made to our medical illustrator, Betsy Ewing, of New Orleans, Louisiana, whose excellent illustrations are a great contribution to this text.

Scott B. Frame, M.D., F.A.C.S.
Norman E. McSwain, Jr., M.D., F.A.C.S.

Contributors

Michael J. Bosse, M.D., F.A.C.S.
Attending Orthopedic Trauma Surgeon
Maryland Institute of Emergency
   Medical Services Systems, and
Associate Professor of Surgery
University of Maryland
Baltimore, Maryland

Scott B. Frame, M.D., F.A.C.S.
Assistant Professor
Division of Trauma/Critical Care
Department of Surgery
University of Tennessee
Graduate School of Medicine
Knoxville, Tennessee

Howard R. Gould, M.D.
Professor of Radiology
Director
Diagnostic Radiology
University of Tennessee
Graduate School of Medicine
Knoxville, Tennessee

Morris D. Kerstein, M.D., F.A.C.S.
Professor and Chairman
Department of Surgery
Hahnamann Medical College
Philadelphia, Pennsylvania

Kimball I. Maull, M.D., F.A.C.S.
Professor of Surgery
University of Maryland School of
   Medicine, and
Director
R. Adams Cowley Shock Trauma Center
Baltimore, Maryland

**Norman E. McSwain, Jr., M.D.,
   F.A.C.S.**
Professor
Department of Surgery
Tulane University School of Medicine
New Orleans, Louisiana

Charles M. Reinert, M.D.
Assistant Professor
Department of Orthopedic Surgery
University of Texas
Southwestern Medical School
Dallas, Texas

R. Mark Saroyan, M.D.
Clinical Assistant Professor
Department of Surgery
University of California at Los Angeles
Torrance, California, and
Staff Surgeon
Kaiser-Permanente Hospital
Rancho Palos Verde, California

**Gregory A. Timberlake, M.D.,
   F.A.C.S.**
Associate Professor
Director
Jon Michael Moore Trauma Center
Department of Surgery
West Virginia University Health
   Sciences Center
Morgantown, West Virginia

Retroperitoneal Trauma

Anatomy of the Retroperitoneum

SCOTT B. FRAME, M.D., F.A.C.S.

The peritoneum creates a closed sac in the male and an open sac in the female (openings at the orifices of the Fallopian tubes). The parietal peritoneum covers the walls of the abdominal cavity and then reflects over the intra-abdominal organs as the visceral peritoneum. Most of the abdominal organs are completely enclosed by peritoneum and receive their blood supply through the vessels traveling in the mesentery. The vessels within the mesentery and structures located between the posterior abdominal wall and the parietal peritoneum constitute the retroperitoneal space. The gastrointestinal tract (GI), of necessity, must enter and exit the peritoneal space, so both ends of the GI tract incorporate sections that are retroperitoneal. Also, some segments of the GI tract do not receive their blood supply through a mesentery and are directly attached to the posterior wall and only covered on their anterior surface by peritoneum. The structures that are considered to be retroperitoneal are listed in Table 1–1.

TERMINAL ESOPHAGUS

The esophagus is about 25 to 30 cm in length, of which only the last 4 to 5 cm lie below the diaphragm and constitute the abdominal or retroperitoneal portion. The esophagus enters the abdomen through the esophageal hiatus of the diaphragm. This opening lies anterior and just to the left of the entrance of the aorta (Fig. 1–1).

Histologically, the esophagus has three coats: muscular, areolar, and mucosal. The muscular coat has two layers, an outer longitudinal and an inner circular. The areolar coat loosely connects the muscular and mucosal layers, but allows a great deal of movement between the two structures. In other words, the mucosa can slide on the muscular coat due to this very loose connection between them. The inner coat of the esophagus is the thick mucosal coat. The mucosa is arranged in longitudinal folds and is of the stratified squamous epithelial variety. The terminal esophagus contains the muscular structures of the lower esophageal sphincter; part of which lies in the thorax, part in the diaphragm, and part in the abdomen. The esophagus has no serosal layer, as is present on the other structures of the alimentary tract. This histologic difference has important consequences in trauma due

Table 1–1   Retroperitoneal Structures

Gastrointestinal tract
   Terminal esophagus
   Duodenum (2nd, 3rd, 4th portions)
   Extrahepatic bile ducts
   Pancreas
   Posterior ascending and descending colon
   Rectum
Genitourinary tract
   Kidneys
   Adrenal glands
   Ureters
   Distal bladder
   Uterus
Vascular system
   Aorta and branches
   Inferior vena cava and tributaries
   Portal vein and tributaries
Musculoskeletal system
   Psoas major and minor
   Iliacus
   Quadratus lumborum
   Thoracoabdominal diaphragm
   Pelvic diaphragm
   Vertebral column
   Pelvic bones
Nervous system
   Spinal cord
   Lumbosacral plexus
   Distal vagal trunks
   Sympathetic and parasympathetic plexus for abdominal viscera, pelvis, lower extremities

to the effects of inflammation and the inability to develop a serositis to help seal small perforations in the esophagus.

The abdominal portion of the esophagus receives its blood supply from a rich anastomotic plexus with vessels from above and from branches of the left gastric artery. An important connection between the portal and systemic venous systems exists in the terminal esophagus where the veins of the esophagus communicate with the left gastric vein. The esophagus is enervated by the sympathetic system, with a plexus lying between the muscular layers and a second plexus lying in the submucosal region.

DUODENUM

The duodenum derives its name from the work of Herophilus of Chalcedon, who lived in Alexandria from 335 to 280 B.C. He named the beginning of the intestines, prior to the beginning of the loops, the "dodekadactilon."[1] This term was derived from the observation that this portion of the alimentary tract had a length equal to the breadth of 12 fingers or 12 thumbs. Galen thought of the duodenum as a structure separate from the stomach and intestine and was merely an organ connecting the stomach to the true intestine.[1] Massa[2]

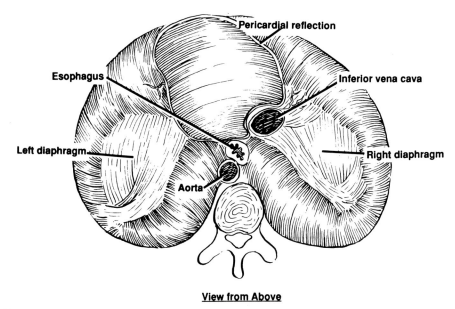

Figure 1–1.   Anatomic relationships of the esophageal hiatus.

(1559) was the first to give a complete description of the alimentary tract from the rectum to the stomach and emphasized the continuity of the alimentary tract.

Embryology

The duodenum is derived from the foregut and the midgut. This embryologic midgut is not to be confused with the surgical midgut (that portion of the alimentary tract supplied by the superior mesenteric artery). The foregut develops into the proximal duodenum and the midgut contributes a portion of the distal duodenum. The C-loop shape of the duodenum arises from the so-called rotation of the duodenum during the sixth week of gestation. In reality, the ventral wall of the duodenum grows and causes the apparent "rotation" of the duodenum, but no torsion of the duodenum actually occurs.

During the early stages of the elongation of the midgut in the yolk sac, two suspensory bands form as thickenings of the dorsal mesentery at the proximal and distal ends of the alimentary tract. The superior band moves into a retroperitoneal position and becomes the suspensory ligament of the duodenum. This band will eventually reach cranially where it inserts on the right medial crus of the diaphragm. During the tenth gestational week, the elongated midgut returns to the abdominal cavity and rotates into its mature position.

The first portion of the duodenum retains both a dorsal and ventral mesentery. However, during the time of the apparent duodenal rotation, the loop becomes fixed in the retroperitoneal space. Therefore, the dorsal mesentery of the second, third, and fourth portions of the duodenum disappears. The remnants of this dorsal mesentery form an avascular plane of loose connective tissue called the fascia of Treitz. It is this plane that is entered during the performance of the Kocher maneuver to mobilize the second and third portions of the duodenum and expose the posterior duodenum and pancreas.

Histology

The duodenal wall consists of a mucosa, a submucosa, a muscularis externa, and an external serosa. The mucosa forms large folds that project into the lumen in a transverse fashion (the valves of Kerckring). These folds are absent in the proximal 2 to 5 cm of the duodenum, forming the duodenal bulb. The mucosa is a columnar epithelium based on a lamina propria of loose connective tissue, bounded by the muscularis mucosa (a thin layer of smooth muscle). The mucosa has villous outgrowths of 0.5 to 1.5 mm in length that have a core of lamina propria and contain muscle fibers from the muscularis mucosa. The lymphatics, capillaries, and nerve fibers run in the core of the villi.

The duodenum is histologically distinct from the remainder of the intestinal tract by the presence of a single feature. There are simple tubular glands between the villi (crypts of Lieberkühn) extending into the lamina propria. The distinctive feature is a submucosa filled with coiled tubular glands that pierce the muscularis mucosa and open into the bottoms of the crypts (Brunner's glands). It is the presence of the glands of Brunner that give the duodenum its characteristic histologic appearance.

The submucosa is bounded by the muscularis externa consisting of two layers. The inner layer is circular smooth muscle and the superficial layer is longitudinal smooth muscle. These two muscular layers form the motor system for peristalsis.

Four sphincters have been described in the duodenum, the actual existence of which is highly controversial.[3] The first sphincter is thought to be located at the distal end of the duodenal bulb. Dysfunction of this sphincter is thought to be responsible for bulbar achalasia and "megabulb." The second is the supra-Vaterian sphincter of Villemin and is located just proximal to the ampulla of Vater. The third is the "Ochsner muscle" and is below the ampulla of Vater, according to Ochsner, who described it in 1906. The last is a sphincter located just proximal to the duodenojejunal flexure and was described by both Ochsner and Villemin. The presence of these structures is dubious, and their clinical significance is probably nil.

Surgical Anatomy

An excellent overview of the surgical anatomy of the duodenum is to be found in the article by Skandalakis et al.[4] The majority of the information covered in this section is from this article.

The junction of the stomach and the duodenum is marked by the thickening of the circular muscle layer to form the pyloric sphincter of the stomach. Distal to this "os pylorus" is the duodenum. Externally, the pylorus is variably marked by the "prepyloric vein of Mayo." The end of the duodenum is the duodenojejunal junction and is marked externally by the attachment of the suspensory ligament of Treitz. There is no other clear line of demarcation at this point.

The first portion of the duodenum is completely covered by peritoneum, whereas all the other portions are covered only on their anterior surfaces and are truly retroperitoneal. The structures responsible for duodenal fixation are the pylorus, superior mesenteric vessels, the ligament of Treitz, and the overlying peritoneum.

The first, or ascending, portion of the duodenum is approximately 5 cm in length. The first half is mobile and the second half is fixed. The duodenum passes cranially from the pylorus to the neck of the gallbladder. Posterior to the first portion of the duodenum lies the common bile duct, portal vein, inferior vena cava, and gastroduodenal artery. It is related anteriorly to the quadrate lobe of the liver, superiorly to the epiploic foramen, and inferiorly to the head of the pancreas.

The second part of the duodenum is also known as the descending duodenum. It is approximately 7.5 cm long and extends from the neck of the gallbladder to the upper border of L4. This portion forms an acute angle with the first part and descends from the neck of the gallbladder. Posterior to this part lies the right kidney, right ureter, right renal vessels, right psoas major, and the lateral edge of the inferior vena cava. Anterior is the right lobe of the liver, transverse colon, and jejunum. The medial, concave surface is related to the head of the pancreas. The lateral surface is related to the ascending colon and the hepatic flexure. At about the midpoint of the second portion, the pancreaticobiliary tract opens onto the posteromedial side at the ampulla of Vater.

The horizontal, or third, portion is about 10 cm long and extends from the right side of L3 or L4 to the left side of the aorta. This part begins about 5 cm to the right of the midline and ends to the left of the vertebral column. Posterior to this portion are the right ureter, right gonadal vessels, right psoas major muscle, inferior vena cava, lumbar vertebral column, and the aorta. The superior mesenteric vessels cross the anterior surface of this portion and, near the distal end, the root of the mesentery of the small bowel crosses over the duodenum. Superior to this part lies the uncinate process of the pancreas, and the pancreaticoduodenal artery lies in a groove at the interface of the duodenum and pancreas. The anterior and inferior surfaces are related to the small bowel, mostly jejunum.

The fourth portion of the duodenum is also an ascending part. It is approximately 2.5 cm long and extends from the left side of the aorta to the left upper margin of L2. It ends at the root of the transverse mesocolon. Posterior to this portion are the left sympathetic trunk, left psoas major muscle, and left renal and gonadal vessels. The upper end of the root of the mesentery attaches anteriorly.

The blood supply of the duodenum arises from branches of both the celiac trunk and the superior mesenteric artery. The first part of the duodenum is supplied by the supraduodenal artery and the posterior superior pancreaticoduodenal branch of the gastroduodenal artery. The remaining duodenum is supplied by an anterior and posterior arcade. Four arteries contribute to these arcades: (1) anterosuperior pancreaticoduodenal arteries (two in number) from the gastroduodenal artery; (2) posterosuperior pancreaticoduodenal artery from the gastroduodenal artery; (3) anteroinferior pancreaticoduodenal artery from the superior mesenteric artery; and (4) posteroinferior pancreaticoduodenal artery from the superior mesenteric artery. Venous drainage follows the arterial arcades, and the blood drains into the superior mesenteric, inferior mesenteric, splenic, and first jejunal veins. Figure 1–2 illustrates the anatomic relationships.

EXTRAHEPATIC BILE DUCTS

The right and left hepatic ducts exit the substance of the liver on the inferior surface and unite to form the common hepatic duct. At the junction of the common hepatic and the cystic duct from the gallbladder, the designation changes to the common bile duct. Other names for this distal duct are the choledochal or, simply, the bile duct. This duct empties into the duodenum in the second portion in common with, or in close proximity to, the main

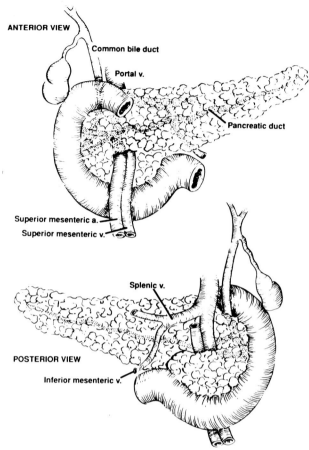

Figure 1–2. Anatomic relationships of the duodenum, pancreas, major ducts, and vessels.

pancreatic duct. The extrahepatic ducts run in the free edge of the lesser omentum, inferiorly to the duodenum, where it courses posterior to this structure and enters, or is enfolded by, the head of the pancreas, and ends at the second portion of the duodenum.

PANCREAS

The pancreas is a gland serving both endocrine and exocrine functions. It is important for the production of digestive enzymes and multiple regulatory hormones, especially insulin for glucose homeostasis.

Embryology

The embryogenesis of the pancreas is closely related to the formation of the duodenum. The pancreas originates as a hollow projection from the dorsal wall of the duodenum, opposite the hepatic diverticulum. This hollow process expands between the two layers of the dorsal mesentery and forms a complicated tubular gland. There is also a ventral pancreatic process that arises in close proximity to the hepatic diverticulum. During the sixth week of gestation, the ventral pancreas and the hepatic diverticulum are carried dorsally around the circumference of the duodenum. As previously pointed out, this rotation comes from the growth of the ventral wall of the duodenum, rather than from an actual rotation. The common duct of the hepatic diverticulum and the ventral pancreatic primordium come to rest adjacent to the dorsal pancreatic process.

These two pancreatic processes fuse, with the ventral process becoming the head and the dorsal becoming the body and tail of the pancreas. The ductal systems of both processes undergo fusion and anastomosis. In most cases the ventral duct combines with the distal portion of the dorsal duct to form the main pancreatic duct (of Wirsung), which opens on the posterior medial wall of the second portion of the duodenum, at the ampulla of Vater. The remnant of the proximal dorsal duct usually persists as the accessory duct (of Santorini) and opens onto the medial wall of the second part of the duodenum, proximal to the ampulla of Vater.

Surgical Anatomy

The pancreas is a pinkish-yellow retroperitoneal organ that lies transversely in the upper abdomen. The head of the gland lies nestled in the C-loop of the duodenum and the tail extends to the hilum of the spleen (Fig. 1–2). The length is from 10 to 15 cm and the weight generally ranges from 60 to 100 gm. It is generally triangular in shape with the apex at the spleen and may be divided into a head (the caudal portion of which is the uncinate process), body, and tail.

The head of the pancreas is the thickest portion of the gland. It lies over the hilum of the right kidney and is just posterior to, and nestled in, the concave portion of the duodenum. It is adherent to the duodenum and envelops the pancreaticoduodenal vessels. The body and tail extend to the left and cranially. Posterior to the gland lie the inferior vena cava, renal veins, vertebral column, aorta, superior mesenteric vessels, left kidney, and left adrenal gland. The splenic vessels normally lie superior to the gland or are at times within the substance of the gland.

Anterior to the pancreas are the stomach, leaves of the transverse mesocolon, transverse colon, liver, and small intestine. The pancreas is separated from the stomach by the lesser peritoneal sac and lies on the transverse duodenum and the duodenojejunal junction. The common bile duct either runs in a groove that may be felt in the posterior portion of the gland or through the substance of the head of the pancreas.

The head of the pancreas shares its blood supply with the duodenum and the remainder of the gland is supplied via anastomosing arcades. The anterior arcade is made up of the anterior superior pancreaticoduodenal artery from the gastroduodenal and the anterior inferior pancreaticoduodenal artery from the superior mesenteric. The posterior arcade is formed from the posterosuperior pancreaticoduodenal artery from the gastroduodenal and the posteroinferior pancreaticoduodenal artery from the superior mesenteric artery. The superior pancreatic artery normally arises from the splenic artery, but may be from the celiac, superior mesenteric, or hepatic arteries. The inferior pancreatic artery generally lies dorsally and inferiorly to the gland and arises from the superior mesenteric and the anterosuperior or anteroinferior pancreaticoduodenal artery. Arterial branches to the body and tail also arise from the splenic and left gastroepiploic arteries. The venous drainage parallels the arterial supply, and the blood drains into the splenic and superior mesenteric veins, which combine beneath the pancreas to form the portal vein.

POSTERIOR ASCENDING AND DESCENDING COLON AND RECTUM

The majority of the large intestine, including the anterior surfaces of the ascending and descending colon, transverse colon, and sigmoid colon, are considered intraperitoneal organs. However, the posterior surfaces of the ascending and descending colon are considered components of the retroperitoneum. The right and left colons are not attached via a mesentery, but rather they are fused to the posterior abdominal wall and the posterior surfaces are devoid of a peritoneal covering. The rectum is the site of exit of the gastrointestinal tract from the peritoneal cavity and is therefore completely retroperitoneal.

Embryology

The primitive alimentary canal is initially attached throughout its extent posteriorly to the primitive notochord via a mesoblastic band from which the common mesentery will be derived. As maturation progresses, the embryologic midgut begins to expand and protrudes out of the abdominal cavity into the yolk stalk. The gut remains attached posteriorly at the future duodenum proximately and the rectum distally. The rectum therefore is a component of the embryologic hindgut.

At about the sixth week of gestation, a lateral diverticulum develops just distal to the vitellointestinal duct. This diverticulum will become the cecum, the boundary between the small and large intestines. The midgut continues to elongate outside the abdominal cavity until the small and large intestines are attached to the vertebral column by a common mesentery. The coils of the small intestine lie to the right of the midline and those of the large intestine lie to the left. By the end of the third month, the intestine is withdrawn back into the abdominal cavity. As this occurs, the gut rotates on itself in a counterclockwise fashion so that the large intestine is carried in front of the small intestine and the cecum comes to rest on the right immediately below the liver. At about the sixth week, the cecum descends farther on the right into the iliac fossa to its adult position. This descent may be arrested at any point and explains the variable position of the cecum in the adult. The mesenteries of the ascending and descending colon disappear and these structures become fixed to the posterior abdominal wall.

Histology

The large intestine has four coats: serous, muscular, areolar, and mucous.

The serous coat is derived from the peritoneum and variably invests the colon. It is absent on the posterior surfaces of the ascending and descending colon. The upper portion of rectum is completely invested, the middle portion is covered only on its anterior surface, and the distal rectum is completely bare.

The muscular coat consists of an external longitudinal and an internal circular muscle layer. In the colon the longitudinal layer does not comprise a uniform investing layer. The muscle is gathered into three flat longitudinal bands, or teniae. These teniae are named for their position on the transverse colon: the tenia libera, tenia omentalis, and tenia mesentericus. At the rectosigmoid junction, the teniae coalesce to form an enveloping longitudinal layer. This histologic change demarcates the beginning of the rectum. The circular muscle layer is continuous throughout the colon and rectum, and in the distal rectum it thickens to form the internal sphincter.

The areolar coat closely connects the muscular and mucosal layers and consists only of connective tissue.

The mucosal coat consists of a muscle layer (the muscularis mucosa), a basement membrane, and the columnar epithelium. The mucous membrane of the colon consists of simple follicles and solitary glands.

Surgical Anatomy

The ascending colon runs up the right gutter of the abdomen from the iliac fossa to the right colic, or hepatic, flexure. This flexure lies just anterior to the right kidney and immediately to the right of the gallbladder on the undersurface of the liver where it rests in an indentation called the impressio colica. The posterior surface is normally fixed to the posterior abdominal wall and the visceral peritoneum reflects back on itself to become the parietal peritoneum lateral to the colonic wall forming the white line of Toldt. Posteriorly, the right colon lies on the quadratus lumborum and transversalis muscles. Anteriorly, the ascending colon is related to the convolutions of the ileum and the abdominal parietes. The ileum enters into the colon at the ileocecal valve and this junction indicates the demarcation between the cecum and the ascending colon. Rarely, the ascending colon does not fuse to the posterior abdominal wall and a small ascending mesocolon remains. In this extremely rare circumstance the posterior ascending colon cannot be considered a retroperitoneal structure.

The descending colon begins where the transverse colon makes a sharp bend posteriorly and inferiorly to form the left, or splenic, colonic flexure. The descending colon passes inferiorly along the lateral border of the left kidney. At the lower margin of the kidney, it makes a medial bend to the lateral edge of the left psoas major muscle, which it follows down to the pelvic brim at the crest of the ileum, where it terminates in the sigmoid flexure. It is fixed in position by the peritoneum, which covers the medial, anterior, and lateral walls, and again reflects back on itself along the lateral wall of the colon to form the left white line of Toldt. Posteriorly, the descending colon lies over the quadratus lumborum and transversalis muscles. The superior end is attached to the diaphragm by a fold of peritoneum, the phrenocolic ligament. The descending colon is smaller in caliber and lies deep to the ascending colon. It more frequently will have a retained mesentery, but this is still a very uncommon occurrence.

The rectum begins at the level of the middle of the sacrum where the sigmoid colon loses its mesentery and the longitudinal muscle layers coalesce to form an enveloping layer. It is approximately 15 cm in length and follows the sacrococcygeal curve. In the upper third it is covered on the anterior and lateral surfaces by peritoneum. The middle third is covered on the anterior surface only and the distal third is devoid of peritoneum entirely.

The rectovesical and rectouterine pouches descend to within 7 to 8 cm and 5 to 6 cm, respectively, of the anus. Below the level of the pouches, the rectum is surrounded by visceral pelvis fascia from the superior fascia of the pelvic diaphragm.

Anteriorly in the male, the rectum is related to coils of the small bowel in the rectovesical pouch above and to the posterior portion of the bladder, prostate, seminal vesicles, and ductus deferentes below. In the female the anterior relationships are to coils of small bowel in the rectouterine pouch above and the posterior portion of the vagina below. Laterally, the rectum is related to the ileum or sigmoid colon. Posteriorly, it is related to the sacrum, coccyx, and pelvic diaphragm.

The blood supply to the colon is dual and is derived from both the superior and inferior mesenteric arteries. The ascending colon is supplied via branches of the ileocolic artery (a terminal branch of the superior mesenteric artery) and the right colic artery (also from the superior mesenteric artery), through a rich anastomotic network. The descending colon is supplied via the left colic artery, a branch of the inferior mesenteric artery. The marginal artery of Drummond connects the two vascular networks from the superior and inferior mesenteric arteries. The rectum is supplied by the superior hemorrhoidal artery (the terminal branch of the inferior mesenteric artery), middle hemorrhoidal artery (from the internal iliac artery), and inferior hemorrhoidal artery (from the external pudendal artery). The venous drainage follows the arterial arcades, and ultimately the blood drains into the inferior and superior mesenteric veins with final drainage into the portal vein. The distal rectum drains into the systemic circulation and the venous plexus present in the rectum marks a connection between the portal and systemic venous systems.

GENITOURINARY TRACT

The kidneys, ureter, and bladder comprise the urinary system. This system is also associated with the terms "renal" and "nephric" from the Latin *ren* and the Greek *nephros*. The urinary system is responsible for maintaining fluid and electrolyte balance in the serum and excreting some of the waste products of metabolism. The ureters connect the kidneys with the bladder and serve as conduits for the transport of urine to the bladder for storage and then excretion. The bladder is also referred to as the vesical, from the Latin *vesica*. The bladder varies in size and shape, depending on the amount of urine contained. The superior surface of the bladder is covered by peritoneum. The remainder of the bladder is bare and, hence, is retroperitoneal. The empty bladder lies almost entirely within the pelvis, but as it fills it ascends into the abdomen. The origins and function of the adrenal glands are distinct from the urinary system but, due to their anatomic proximity, will be considered in this section. Injury to any of these structures may cause a retroperitoneal hematoma and a diagnostic quandary at exploration.

Embryology

The kidneys and ureters are formed from the primitive "intermediate cell mass," which differentiates into the wolffian duct. Further differentiation occurs as the wolffian duct forms many convoluted tubules and eventually encloses a tuft, or glomerulus, of forming capillaries. The ureters are formed from a protrusion from the posterior end of the wolffian duct.

The bladder forms from a dilation of the second part of the allantois. By the end of the second month of gestation, this dilation enlarges into a spindle-shaped cavity that persists as the bladder.

The adrenal glands form from two different sources. The medullary portion of the glands is derived from the tissues forming the sympathetic ganglia of the abdomen. The cortical portion is of mesoblastic origin and forms from an outgrowth of the upper part of the wolffian body. The two portions fuse to lose their distinct character and form the final gland.

Histology

The histologic characteristics of the renal system and the adrenal glands are too complex for an adequate description to be undertaken here. The reader is referred to standard histology texts for an in-depth discussion of this topic.

Surgical Anatomy

The kidneys are reddish-brown organs covered by a thin, fibromuscular capsule. Each has an anterior and posterior surface, upper and lower pole, and medial and lateral borders. The medial border contains an indentation where the vessels enter and exit and the ureter emerges. Each contains a pale cortical region and a darker medulla. The kidneys lie obliquely along the vertebral column on top of the psoas major muscle (Fig. 1–3).

The upper pole of each kidney is covered by an adrenal gland. Anteriorly, the right

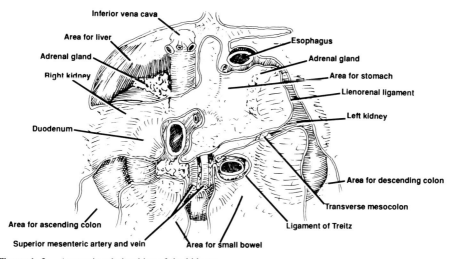

Figure 1–3.   Anatomic relationships of the kidneys.

kidney is associated with the duodenum, ascending colon, right colonic flexure, and small intestine. The right kidney forms an indentation on the undersurface of the liver called the impressio renalis. The left kidney is related on its anterior surface to the spleen, descending colon, left colonic flexure, stomach, pancreas, and small intestine. On the posterior surface, the kidneys are related to the 12th rib, diaphragm, psoas major, quadratus lumborum, and transversus abdominis. The lateral border is convex and is directed outward and backward, toward the posterolateral abdominal wall. On the left side, the upper portion of the lateral border is in contact with the spleen. The medial border is concave and is directed forward and a little downward. The lower pole extends down to within 2 inches of the iliac crest. The right kidney normally lies slightly lower than the left, due to the presence of the liver on the right.

At the hilum, the relative positions of the structures as they pass into and out of the kidney are: the vein is in front, the artery in the middle, and the ureter behind and toward the lower part of the hilum. The kidney is surrounded by a distinct investment of fibrous tissue, Gerota's fascia, which forms a firm, smooth covering. This layer may be easily stripped off.

The renal arteries arise as direct branches off the aorta, and the right renal artery passes behind the vena cava. The left renal artery originates from the aorta just distal to the superior mesenteric artery and branches off the lateral wall of the aorta. The right renal artery takes off of the opposite aortic wall, just distal to the takeoff of the left. The left renal vein is longer than the right and passes anterior to the aorta. This is an important landmark because the takeoff of the left renal artery normally lies just beneath the left renal vein as it passes over the aorta. The left adrenal gland is also drained by the left renal vein, whereas the right adrenal has its own draining vein. The left vein also has tributaries from the left gonad, diaphragm, and body wall. Both renal veins drain straight into the lateral borders of the vena cava.

The adrenal, or suprarenal, glands are paired endocrine organs located above the kidneys. The glands consist of two distinct endocrine organs, the cortex and medulla. The glands are surrounded by renal fascia and lie on the superomedial aspect of the front of the kidney. The right gland lies in contact with the undersurface of the liver behind the inferior vena cava. The left gland is related in front to the lesser sac, splenic artery, and pancreas. Both glands lie on the diaphragm. The arterial supply to the glands is variable and comes from the inferior phrenic, renal arteries, or the aorta. The venous drainage goes directly to the inferior vena cava on the right and to the renal vein on the left.

The ureter is a distensible tube connecting the kidney with the bladder. It is abdominal for one half of its course and pelvic for the second half. It runs in the retroperitoneum for its entire length. It commences as a dilation at the renal pelvis posterior to the renal vessels and descends on the surface of the psoas major muscle. The ureters pass anterior to the iliac vessels as they descend into the pelvis, constituting an important landmark. They continue down the lateral wall of the pelvis and turn medially to reach the bladder. In the female the ureters turn downward, forward, and medially at the level of the ischial spine and pass beneath the uterine vessels, about 2 cm from the cervix. At this point, they are in danger of damage during the course of a hysterectomy. The ureters normally lie medial to the ascending and descending colon. The ureters lie posterior to the ileum on the right and the sigmoid flexure of the colon on the left.

The ureters are supplied with blood via an investing plexus of vessels derived from branches of the renal, gonadal, internal iliac, and inferior vesical arteries.

The empty bladder is pyramidal in shape and is described as having four sides: superior, right and left inferolateral, and posterior (or the base). The superior surface and the upper part of the base are covered by peritoneum. The peritoneal relationships of the bladder are important in trauma because they determine whether a bladder rupture is intraperitoneal or retroperitoneal. Posteriorly, the peritoneum forms the rectovesical (or uterovesical) pouch. The superior surface is related to the small bowel, sigmoid colon and/or cecum, and the body of the uterus in the female. The inferolateral surfaces are associated with the retropubic space, which contains a fat pad, and the pelvic venous plexus. The base faces downward and posterior and is in contact with the seminal vesicles, ductus deferentes, and rectum in the male, and the vagina and supravaginal cervix in the female.

The apex of the bladder is connected to the umbilicus by the median umbilical ligament, which is a remnant of the urachus. There are also connections to the umbilicus via the paired medial umbilical ligaments, which are remnants of the obliterated umbilical arteries. The main portion of the bladder is termed the "body" and the lowest portion, the "neck." The neck is attached to the pelvic diaphragm and, in the male, is continuous with the prostate. The trigone of the bladder consists of the orifices of the paired ureters and the internal orifice of the urethra. The blood supply to the bladder is via the superior and inferior vesical arteries, which are branches of the internal iliac arteries. The veins drain into the internal iliac veins.

The urethra is a fibromuscular tube that conducts urine from the bladder to the exterior. It begins at the neck of the bladder and traverses the pelvic and urogenital diaphragms. It is about 4 cm in length in the female and 20 cm in the male. In the female it is fused to the anterior wall of the vagina and ends between the clitoris and the vagina. The male urethra consists of three parts: the prostatic, membranous, and spongy. The membranous part descends from the prostate to the bulb of the penis and is surrounded by the sphincter urethrae. It is this portion of the male urethra that is prone to injury during catheterization or as a result of pelvic fractures.

VASCULAR SYSTEM

The vascular system in the retroperitoneum consists of the aorta and its branches, vena cava and its tributaries, and the portal vein and its tributaries. Injury to these structures carries the potential for massive hemorrhage. This massive blood loss is the principal cause of early death in the trauma patient, and injuries to other structures carry much higher mortalities when there is an associated vascular injury.

Embryology

The abdominal aorta rises from the fusion of the paired aorta arising from the simple tubular heart. This fusion begins in the thorax and proceeds caudally. The umbilical arteries rise after the fusion occurs and initially appear as almost a bifurcation of the now fused primitive aorta. The common and internal iliac arteries are formed by the proximal remnants of the umbilical arteries. The remainder of the umbilical arteries become obliterated at birth except for the portion that gives rise to the superior vesical arteries. The external iliac and femoral arteries are formed from a small branch of the umbilical artery given off near the origin of the umbilical vessels. The visceral arteries are formed from the branches of the two primitive aortas that supply the omphalomesenteric vessels to the yolk sac.

The development of the venous system is more complex and involves the formation of two different groups of vessels, the visceral and the parietal. The visceral veins form from the two vitelline, or omphalomesenteric, veins, returning blood from the yolk sac, and the two umbilical veins, returning blood from the placenta. The portal vein is formed from the fusion of the two vitelline veins, which receive branches from the alimentary tract.

The cardinal veins form in the lower trunk and return blood from the parietes and the wolffian bodies. The blood from the lower limbs is returned via the iliac veins to the cardinal veins. The right cardinal vein becomes the dominant vessel as transverse branches carry the blood from the left iliac and renal veins to the right cardinal. Up to the level of the renal veins, the right cardinal vein develops into the inferior vena cava. The vena cava above the level of the renal veins forms from a small vessel that originally lies between the two primitive kidneys. This vessel gradually enlarges to become the upper portion of the inferior vena cava, emptying into the heart.

Surgical Anatomy

Aorta

The abdominal aorta begins at the aortic hiatus of the diaphragm as the vessel passes from the thorax into the abdomen. The diaphragmatic hiatus lies at about the level of the 12th thoracic vertebra. The aorta descends anterior to the vertebral bodies and ends at the bifurcation into the left and right common iliac arteries, at about the level of the fourth lumbar vertebra. The branches of the abdominal aorta, as in their embryologic development, are divided into parietal and visceral branches. All of the parietal branches are paired except for the median sacral artery, which arises in the midline at the aortic bifurcation. The remainder of the vessels arise from the lateral walls of the aorta. There is a pair of inferior phrenic and four pairs of lumbar arteries given off by the abdominal aorta. Each common iliac artery bifurcates into an internal and external branch. The external iliac artery proceeds out of the abdomen to the lower extremities, giving off the inferior epigastric and deep circumflex iliac arteries prior to exiting (Fig. 1–4).

The internal iliac artery supplies most of the blood to the pelvis. The parietal branches of the internal iliac are the iliolumbar, lateral sacral, obturator, superior and inferior gluteal, and internal pudendal arteries. The visceral branches are the umbilical, superior and inferior vesical, uterine, vaginal, and middle rectal arteries.

The majority of the visceral branches of the abdominal aorta are unpaired and arise from the anterior surface of the vessel. The two sets of paired vessels are the gonadal and renal arteries. The gonadal arteries arise below the level of the renal arteries and descend on top of the psoas major muscles. The left renal artery is short and passes directly into the kidney. The right renal artery is longer and passes posterior to the vena cava before entering the kidney. The superior and inferior mesenteric arteries and celiac trunk are unpaired and supply blood to the abdominal organs.

The celiac trunk is the first branch on the anterior surface of the aorta and arises just below the diaphragmatic hiatus. It branches into the left gastric, splenic, and common

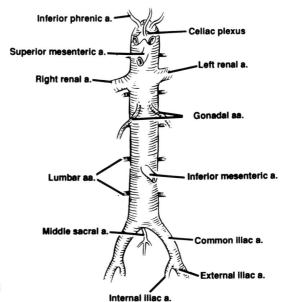

Figure 1–4. The branches of the abdominal aorta.

hepatic arteries. The left gastric artery courses along the lesser curvature of the stomach and anastomoses with the right gastric artery. The splenic artery courses along the superior border of the pancreas and gives off pancreatic branches, the left gastroepiploic artery, and the short gastric arteries prior to entering the spleen. The common hepatic artery runs to the right along the upper border of the head of the pancreas, giving off several pancreatic branches. At the level of the duodenum, it divides into the proper hepatic, right gastric, and gastroduodenal arteries. The proper hepatic artery divides into the right and left hepatic arteries before entering the substance of the liver. The cystic artery normally arises from the right hepatic artery. The right gastric artery runs along the lesser curvature where the anastomosis with the left gastric artery occurs. The gastroduodenal artery gives off the posterosuperior pancreaticoduodenal artery and branches into the anterosuperior pancreaticoduodenal and right gastroepiploic arteries.

The superior mesenteric artery emerges in front of the uncinate process of the pancreas and passes anterior to the duodenum. It supplies the surgical midgut: the bowel from the middle of the duodenum to the left part of the transverse colon. Its branches include the inferior pancreaticoduodenal, ileocolic, right colic, and middle colic arteries. It also gives rise to the jejunal and ileal arteries supplying the small intestine.

The inferior mesenteric artery arises just proximal to the aortic bifurcation. It supplies the hindgut: the large intestine from the left transverse colon, distally. Its branches include the left colic and sigmoid arteries, and it terminates in the superior rectal (hemorrhoidal) artery.

Portal Vein

The blood returning from the stomach and intestines is carried by the portal venous system to the liver and thence to the vena cava via the hepatic veins. In this fashion the nutrients absorbed from the gastrointestinal tract are taken immediately to the liver for processing prior to entering the systemic circulation. The portal vein is formed posterior to the neck of the pancreas by the merging of the superior mesenteric and splenic veins (Fig. 1–5). The inferior mesenteric vein joins the splenic vein prior to its junction with the superior mesenteric vein. The left gastric and prepyloric veins join the portal vein after its creation. The mesenteric venous system parallels the arterial system up to the point of the formation of the unique portal venous system. The portal vein enters the hepatoduodenal ligament and ascends to divide at the porta hepatis into right and left branches.

There are five important areas of anastomosis between the portal venous system and the systemic circulation:

1. The inferior mesenteric vein and the inferior vena cava and its tributaries
2. Gastric veins and the superior vena cava and its tributaries
3. Retroperitoneal veins and the caval system
4. Paraumbilical and subcutaneous veins
5. Superior and middle hemorrhoidal veins, and inferior hemorrhoidal vein

Inferior Vena Cava

The inferior vena cava is formed by the union of the iliac veins at the level of the fifth lumbar vertebra. It ascends in the retroperitoneum to the right of the aorta and traverses the central

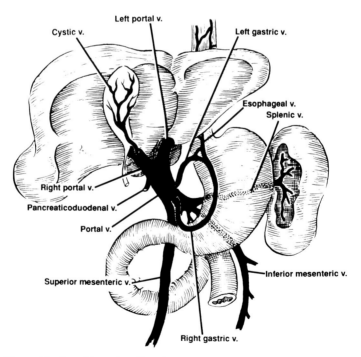

Figure 1–5.   The portal vein and its major tributaries.

tendon of the diaphragm to empty into the right atrium. The usual tributaries of the vena cava are the common iliac, right gonadal, renal, adrenal, inferior phrenic, lumbar, and hepatic veins. Most of these are paired veins except for the gonadal and hepatic veins. The right gonadal vein empties directly into the vena cava, whereas the left drains into the corresponding renal vein. The hepatic veins enter the vena cava just caudad to the diaphragm and are behind the liver, making surgical exposure and control extremely difficult. There are normally three main hepatic veins, although there is often a fourth. These include the right, middle, and left veins and, variably, a vein from the caudate lobe. The inferior vena cava lies on the psoas major muscle for most of its length and runs just to the right of the aorta throughout the retroperitoneum. The iliac veins are deep to the arteries and the left renal vein passes over the aorta to reach the left kidney. The gonadal vessels cross over the ureters at the level of the pelvic brim.

DIAPHRAGM

A detailed description of the anatomy of the diaphragm is included in Chapter 14 and will not be repeated here.

PELVIS

The pelvis derives its name from the Latin term for basin, which the structure closely resembles. It is stronger than either the cranial or thoracic cavities. It forms a bony ring that is interposed between the spine, which it supports, and the lower extremities, upon which it rests (Fig. 1–6).

The pelvic girdle is made up of four bones: two innominate, the sacrum, and the coccyx. The two innominate bones (also called the hip bones or the os coxae) are made up in childhood of three separate bones that fuse during adolescent development at the acetabulum. These three bones are the ilium, ischium, and pubis. Each contributes to the formation of the acetabulum, with the superior third being from the ilium, the anterior third from the pubis, and posteroinferior third from the ischium. The two innominate bones articulate anteriorly in the midline at the symphysis pubis and posteriorly with the sacrum. The sacrum, in turn, articulates inferiorly with the coccyx.

The pelvis is divided anatomically and functionally into a true and a false pelvis. The division plane runs through the upper symphysis pubis, iliopectineal and arcuate lines, and the promontory of the sacrum. This oblique plane forms the pelvic inlet and separates the false pelvis above from the true pelvis below. The true pelvis contains the organs of reproduction, and through it passes portions of the urinary and gastrointestinal tracts, and major vessels and nerves to the lower extremities. The false pelvis is actually part of the abdominal cavity and contains intra-abdominal structures.

The major function of the pelvis is to provide support to the spine. In the erect individual the weight-bearing forces are transmitted from the upper femoral bones to the acetabula and then through thick rings on the ilia called the "arcuate lines." These rings curve superiorly and posteriorly to the sacroiliac joints and then into the spinal column through the sacrum. In the sitting position the weight is transferred through the sacroiliac joints into the ilia and down to the ischial tuberosities, forming the ischiosacral arch.

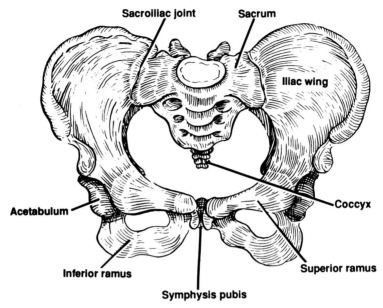

Figure 1–6.   The anatomic features of the pelvis in anteroposterior projection.

The pelvis contains a rich network of arteries and veins. The arteries are supplied by the internal iliac (hypogastric) artery and consist of the parietal and visceral branches, as outlined earlier in this chapter. The venous system forms a rich pelvic plexus that drains into a venous network corresponding to the arterial system and eventually drains into the internal iliac (hypogastric) vein, which lies deep to the artery. The highly vascular nature of the true pelvis is the reason for the massive hemorrhage associated with some pelvic fractures, leading to the high mortality of these injuries.

REFERENCES

1.   Galen C: *On the usefulness of the parts of the body*. (Translated by May MT.) Ithaca: Cornell University Press, 1968.
2.   Massa N: Liber introductorius anatomiae (1536). In Bindoni, Pasini (eds): *Studies in Pre-Vesalian Anatomy*. (Translated by Lind LR.) Philadelphia: American Philosophical Society, 1975.
3.   Didio LJA, Anderson MC: *The "Sphincters" of the Digestive System*. Baltimore: Williams & Wilkins, 1968.
4.   Skandalakis JE, Skandalakis LJ, Colborn GL, et al: The duodenum. Surgical anatomy. *Am Surg* 1989;55: 291–298.

2

Kinematics of Retroperitoneal Trauma

NORMAN E. McSWAIN, JR., M.D., F.A.C.S.

A major component of vehicular trauma and falls that affect the retroperitoneal organs is a sudden change of direction and change in velocity of the victim, producing shear injuries. The moving body and its support structures suddenly decrease their motion. The organs that are attached firmly to the supporting structures of the body rapidly stop also. Those portions of these organs that are not firmly attached continue in motion (Newton's first law of motion) until the attachments to the solid structures reduce their motion. The shear forces that develop between the moving component and the fixed component can produce tears that result in injury. The most obvious retroperitoneal structure affected by such a mechanism of injury is the kidney. The aorta is firmly fixed to the vertebral column. The kidney is held in place by the fat and fascia. Continued forward motion of the kidneys, after the vertebral column and aorta have stopped, stretches the vascular attachments to the kidney. The pedicle can be torn free or stretched to the point of producing intimal damage without external signs.

The opposite effect occurs if the body is rapidly accelerated and the organ is pulled along, such as occurs in a lateral impact collision.

Falls from a height of 20 feet or greater produce multiple deceleration and crush type injuries. Such injuries may be more common in the retroperitoneal area than in the free abdominal cavity.[1]

Although one would think that penetrating trauma is very different from blunt trauma, actually the same physical laws affect both and produce similar injury at the time of the actual impact. Penetrating trauma exerts force over a small area of the body and the tissue resistance is not enough to prevent the skin from being penetrated. Also usually associated with penetrating trauma is a permanent injury that can be easily seen.[2,3]

This chapter will explain both of these types of trauma and demonstrate both their similarities and differences.

PHYSICAL LAWS

Several physical laws are important to understand, since the reactions and results that they describe directly impact on the injury to the patient.[4]

Newton's first law of motion: An object in motion or an object at rest tends to remain in that state until acted on by some outside force.

Newton's law of energy: Energy can neither be created nor destroyed, but it can be changed in form.

Potential energy:

$$KE = \frac{M \times V^2}{2}$$

where KE = kinetics energy, M = mass, and V = velocity.

Force: Force is equal to mass times acceleration (deceleration).

$$F = MA$$

The results of these laws on the patient can be simplistically considered. Once an object obtains a given velocity (energy), to change that velocity (energy) some other energy force must act on the moving body. To reduce the moving body's motion back to zero, an amount of energy equal to that contained by the body in motion must be imparted to it. As previously stated, energy can be neither created nor destroyed, it must be absorbed. Energy absorption usually produces tissue damage. The force applied to an object in motion, or the force necessary to stop an object's motion, is related to the object's mass and to the rate of acceleration or deceleration. The kinetic energy contained by any object in motion is affected by the velocity of the moving object in a far greater manner than the object's weight, or mass, although mass cannot be discounted regarding the effect it has on the final amount of injury. Kocher described the four components that played a part of this mechanism of energy dissipation in his book published in 1880 (*Ueber Schusswunden. Experimentelle Untersuchungen ueber die Wirkungsweise der Midernen Klein-Gerwehr-Geschosse*).[5] These are heat, energy exchange to impart motion to the impacted tissues, crush damage to the tissues that produces a permanent cavity, and deformation of the moving body.

Both penetrating and blunt trauma injure a patient by moving the tissue particles away from their original position to another position. This change produces tearing, stretching, or crushing of the tissue. Tissue injury can be looked at from one of these three conditions. Compressed tissue is crushed, either partially or totally. Partial compression merely damages the tissue, whereas crush destroys it. In the same manner, movement of the tissue away from the point of impact can merely stretch the tissue or it can totally separate it from its origin.

Cavitation: Particle motion away from the point of impact results in either stretch, tear, compression, or crush of the tissue and produces a cavity in that tissue. Such cavitation can either be temporary or permanent. The size of the temporary cavity depends on the amount of energy exchange that occurs within a tissue, whereas the size of the permanent cavitation depends on the amount of elastic tissue or rebound present as well as the frontal area of the impacting object. Tissue that has only a minimal amount of elasticity to produce rebound leaves a temporary cavity almost the exact same size as the permanent cavity (e.g., bone). A large amount of elastic tissue results in a permanent cavity that is far smaller than a temporary one (e.g., blood). Example: A steel drum hit with a baseball bat leaves a visible "cavity" (permanent) at the point of impact. A foam rubber drum hit with the same force develops a temporary cavity that disappears when the bat is removed. Inside the body, cavitation within a muscle tends to produce a small permanent cavity, whereas one within bone tends to produce a large permanent cavity.

As a general rule, the temporary cavity following penetrating trauma tends to occur laterally away from the point of injury, whereas in blunt trauma it tends to be directly away from the impact point.

ENERGY EXCHANGE

The amount of energy exchange that occurs depends on the density of the medium that is impacted, the area of the frontal projection of the moving body, and the energy (mass and velocity) of the moving body. Density is defined as a number of particles per unit volume of that medium or tissue. The surface area (frontal projection) of the impacting object in turn influences the number of particles hit by the moving object: The more particles that are hit, the greater the energy exchange that will occur between the two bodies. Since energy is neither created nor destroyed, the moving body must impart its energy of motion to the stable particles of the impacted tissue. This will reduce the speed of the moving body. If and when all of the energy is exchanged, the moving object will stop.

Any mechanism that changes the frontal area of the projectile will influence the number of particles hit and therefore the energy exchange (Fig. 2–1). The area of impact or frontal projection (area) of the moving object is influenced by three factors: shape, tumble, and fragmentation.

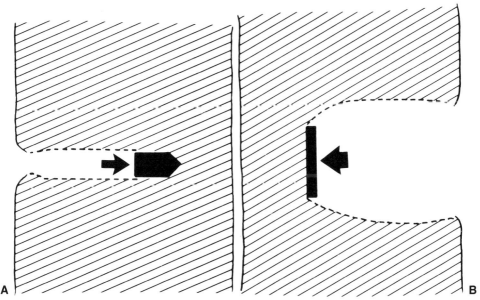

Figure 2–1. Change in the frontal area will significantly alter the number of tissue particles impacted on and therefore the amount of energy exchange that occurs between the moving object and the patient.

Shape

The frontal projection or surface area can be changed by expanding this area. Such a change can occur if the projectile mushrooms on initial contact with the human tissue. The effect that this expansion can have was discovered by the British in their conflicts in India in the latter part of the 1800s. In 1895, their manufacturing facility in India at Dum-Dum began to produce projectiles that would deform to enlarge the frontal size. Thus, the name "Dum-Dum bullet" was born. The missile changes its aerodynamic shape from one that meets very little resistance as it passes through the air to one that encounters a large number of tissue particles. Such ballistic changes can allow a missile (projectile) to retain most of the energy imparted to it when it left the muzzle of the gun en route to the tissue to a shape that allows exchange of most of that energy onto the tissue as it traverses it (Fig. 2–2). These

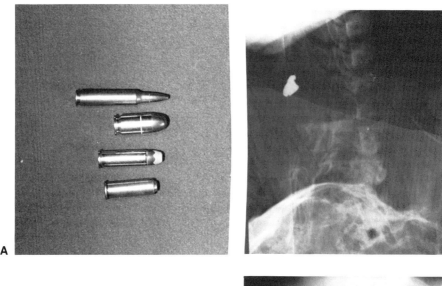

A

B

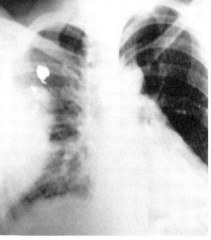

C

Figure 2–2. A very streamlined shape of a missile that impacts on very few particles en route to the target minimally reduces the energy of the missile. If the shape drastically alters at the time of impact, then energy exchange becomes much greater, producing significant damage to the patient.

projectiles were considered to be "inhumane" for warfare and were outlawed by the signatories at the peace conference at The Hague.

Tumble

A missile or a projectile whose longitudinal axis is at 90° to its path of travel will have a greater frontal area than will the same projectile if its longitudinal axis is in the same direction as its path. It is therefore advantageous for a missile to travel in a straight line with a longitudinal axis lined up with the direction of travel en route to a target, but to tumble and present a 90° side view immediately on impact (Fig. 2–3). The Russian AK 74 has much more destructive potential than the same size, weight, and velocity of the AK 47 by increasing the rate of tumble.[6]

Fragmentation

A projectile that breaks up into many small pieces will obviously impact on more tissue particles than will the missile that does not break up and simply bores a hole through an object (Fig. 2–4). The ultimate in fragmentation is represented by the shotgun. The defect of the shotgun, however, is in its effective distance. Close range, the energy exchange from the multiple pellets is great and produces much tissue damage. Because these multiple projectiles try to spread apart immediately on leaving the muzzle of the shotgun, there tends to be a greater energy exchange with the air while en route to the victim, thus dissipating the energy of motion if the distance is great between the weapon and its target.[7–9]

The science of ballistics can be analyzed to make the projectile achieve the goal of its producer.[10,11] Although there are variations, this can be broken down into three separate groups. A hunter wishes his animal to be killed as quickly as possible to reduce the amount of tracking necessary to find the animal and retrieve the meat to eat. A law enforcement officer, on the other hand, is interested in stopping the perpetrator immediately so that the assailant will not have an opportunity to provide further threat to the officer or the bystanders. Whether the patient lives or dies is of no immediate consequence. In a military situation, it is not desirable to kill the combatant. A dead combatant can be replaced by one individual. It will require up to six people to replace and care for the injured as well as use up supplies and other valuable resources such as transportation. Therefore, the cost to the enemy is greater when the opponents are injured and not killed.

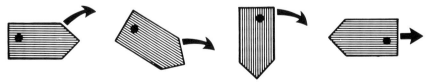

Figure 2–3. Alteration of the position of the missile from small frontal area to large side area (tumble) increases the impact area and the number of tissue particles involved.

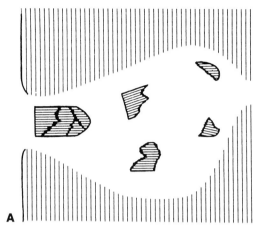

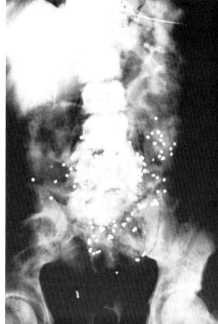

Figure 2–4.   **A**: If a missile breaks up into many pieces, each individual component not only increases the area of impact, but also increases the size of impact and the possible number of organs injured. **B**: The ultimate in fragmentation is the shotgun.

B

BLUNT TRAUMA

In a vehicular collision the pedestrian or occupant of the car is impacted on by an object whose large frontal projection does not crush enough tissue to penetrate, but nonetheless creates a cavity within the body and therefore produces injury.

Vehicular trauma can be divided into vehicle versus vehicle, vehicle versus immovable object, vehicle versus pedestrian, and motocyclist versus immovable object.[4] In all forms of vehicle crashes, similar forces must be considered. The vehicle and its occupant are traveling at the same rate of speed, but with different energy potential (mass difference between vehicle and the occupant). The vehicle impacts on an object and deforms to absorb the energy of its velocity and mass. In vehicle versus pedestrian and motorcyclist versus object, the patient is not surrounded by a structure that aids in energy absorption and therefore all energy is transferred to the patient.

The passenger compartment of an automobile tends to provide some protection from injury via energy absorption, but the patient is nonetheless moving at the same rate as the vehicle just prior to impact. The vehicle suddenly slows, but the occupant does not. The occupant is now traveling at a different rate of speed (much faster) than the passenger compartment. If the occupant is buckled tightly with a good occupant restraint system, then he tends to slow at the same rate as the car and does not impact on the inside of the compartment.

Finally, the organs of the victim's body remain in motion even though the carrier (victim's body) has come to rest. Deformation of the body cavity occurs and organ crush and organ shear result. Vehicular collisions such as this can be divided into five categories that produce different kinds of injury patterns, depending on the direction of motion of the vehicle.

Frontal Impact

As a vehicle stops its forward motion, the unrestrained occupant continues to travel in the frontal direction until he is either ejected from the car or until some part of the body hits an interior component of the car. The body can travel forward in one of two different direction patterns.

Down and Under

The lower extremity is the lead point in the human projectile. The first point of contact with the interior of the car is either the floor pan or pedals by the feet, or the dash by the knees. The feet will frequently twist off the brake pedal, creating a fracture dislocation of the ankle. The leg traveling forward will impact on the dashboard with either the patella, the tibia, or the femur (Fig. 2–5).

Once the lower part of the body stops its forward motion, the torso will rotate in a forward direction, impacting on either the dashboard or the steering column. Deceleration of the abdominal organs occurs as a part of this first motion. Depending on the area impacted on, the energy distribution may be into the abdomen, the chest, or the face.

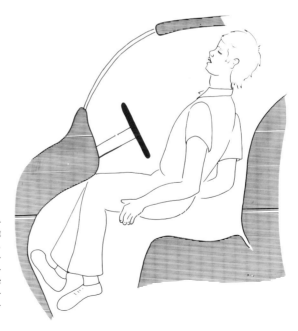

Figure 2–5. The knee moving forward impacting on the dash will suddenly stop that portion of the body and ultimately the torso. The continued momentum of the organs inside the abdominal cavity and the retroperitoneal area is absorbed as shear of these organs from their attachments to the abdominal cavity or to other retroperitoneal structures.

Up and Over

In this pattern the head becomes the lead point of the human projectile. The head will either impact on the top of the passenger compartment or the windshield.

The damage to the various body cavities will produce compression injuries, shear injuries, or a combination of both.

Compression

First the abdominal cavity will compress and then fracture the solid organs, rupture the abdominal cavity itself (like a closed paper bag suddenly subjected to compressive force), or any of the hollow organs such as a gallbladder, urinary bladder, or closed component of the gastrointestinal tract. The urinary bladder and ureter can rupture in the free peritoneal cavity or in the retroperitoneal space.

Shear

Shear injuries can affect the bowel mesentery or the pedicles of the spleen or kidney where the vessels are fixed to the aorta while the organs remain in motion. The liver can also be subject to this force as it travels downward with the right and left halves following separate pathways around the ligamentum teres.

Lateral Impact

A lateral impact changes the direction of motion of the occupants inside the car from frontal motion to lateral motion. The injuries to the patient can be approximated by looking at the injury to the vehicle. Lateral compression of the vehicle crushing in the door will produce a similar pattern on the side of the chest of the unrestrained occupant. The energy exchange to the occupant is at three areas; the lateral chest wall that inwardly compresses the ribs and produces compression to the lung, liver, or spleen; the pelvic structure will fracture either through the impact on the femur near the greater trochanter, forcing the head of the femur into the acetabulum or directly into the wing of the ileum itself; and rotation and lateral flexion of the cervical spine. These lateral movements produce shear and compression injuries similar to those described for a frontal impact, except they will affect the organ on the side of injury (spleen or kidney) far more than the similar structure on the opposite side. The thoracic aorta and shear injuries at the arch are certainly a part of the lateral impact collision and may be more frequent with lateral impact than with a frontal impact.

Rear Impact Collision

The car impacted from the rear is rapidly accelerated forward. Everything attached to the car will rapidly accelerate with the vehicle. Those parts of the occupant that are in contact with one of these structures will also be rapidly accelerated. Those body parts not in contact will only change forward velocities when their attachments to the occupant pull them forward.

The frequent second component of this collision sequence begins when the vehicle moves forward and impacts on the vehicle in front of it. The occupant collision then becomes a frontal impact. Frontal forces are far less in this form of collision than when the frontal impact is the first event. The amount of energy exchange that occurred can be judged by damage to both the front and rear of the vehicle.

Rotation

Rotational injuries occur as one part of the car hits an immovable object or is hit by another vehicle and rotates around a pivot point (Fig. 2–6). The injuries produced are combination frontal and lateral injuries associated with initial point of impact and the direction in which the vehicle rotated. The direction of rotation and the change of velocity can be determined by the condition at the scene.

Multiple Vehicle Collisions

In most collisions that involve more than one car, the kinematics are different for each vehicle. Therefore the patients must be evaluated based on the vehicle they were in, including the direction of impact and the velocity change, rather than evaluating everyone as if they were all in the same automobile.

An easy rule to use in vehicle collisions is that the unrestrained patient is damaged in the same place and with the same energy as the vehicle in which the patient was riding.

OCCUPANT RESTRAINT SYSTEMS

Occupant restraint systems initially were the six point suspensions still used today in racing vehicles. This system has proven to be very effective and is a major reason why both stock and sport car racing is as safe as it is. These safety restraint devices, along with the reinforced supports on the inside of the car that provide excellent protection from intrusion,

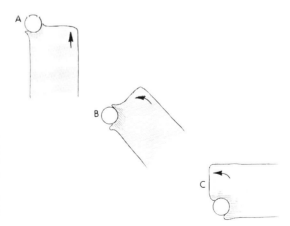

Figure 2–6. When the impact is not centered, rotation occurs around the impact point. For example, when the left front quarter panel hits an immovable object and the right front quarter panel continues to move, then the patient inside the passenger compartment follows a similar pathway, combining both frontal and lateral impact injuries.

significantly reduce injuries in this sport. Less effective devices such as air bags are not used in racing vehicles.

Acceptance of such safety devices by auto drivers in the United States has been less than universal. The philosophical reasons for this nonacceptance range from lack of comfort and efficient restraints available in United States cars compared with foreign cars; lack of adequate education of drivers; and desire for personal freedom. The reasons are inappropriate items for discussion here. Suffice it to say that seat belt usage in the United States, without mandatory seat belt legislation and adequate enforcement of such legislation, is less than 50%. For this reason, passive safety devices such as knee bars, automatic seat belts, and now air bags have come into use. There are defects in each system. Airbags are effective in only 70% of collisions (headlight to headlight collisions). They are not effective in side impact collisions, rollovers, or when there is a second collision. The physician dealing with these patients, however, should be aware that such defects exist and be able to anticipate the injury patterns when air bags are used alone rather than as a supplement to proper belts. Airbags are certainly a supplemental protection device, but must be used with at least a lap belt.

An appropriately placed lap belt is at a 45° angle to the floor below the anterosuperior iliac spine, above the femur, and tight enough to remain in that position. If the lap belt is not tight enough and is allowed to ride above the anterosuperior iliac spine in a frontal impact, forward motion of the vertebral column is halted across the lap belt. Increased intra-abdominal pressure and compression of the soft tissues, similar to a steering column injury, can result to the abdominal organs. In addition, as the pelvis continues to move forward and the upper torso moves forward at the same time, compression fractures at the T-12, L1, and L2 are produced.

SPECIFIC ORGAN INJURIES

The organs of the retroperitoneum are susceptible to compression damage from blunt trauma. Any portion of the passenger compartment can become a relative immovable object in relation to the continued motion of the occupant. As an example, the steering column stops the forward motion of the anterior abdominal wall. The continued momentum of the vertebral column and posterior abdominal wall from behind compresses the retroperitoneal structures. The pancreas, duodenum, spleen, and kidney are vulnerable to being compressed in this fashion.

Another mechanism of importance in producing retroperitoneal trauma occurs during the lateral impact collision. Impact against the door of the occupant's car during an intersectional collision changes the direction of the vehicle motion from forward to lateral. The lateral motion of the unrestrained victim begins only when impacted on by the door of his own car. Two types of forces occur. First, the change in direction of the vehicle motion from forward to lateral impacts on the occupant and, second, intrusion of the door into the passenger as the door itself absorbs energy and is deformed. The restrained occupant will begin his or her lateral motion at the same time that the car moves. This reduces the impact on the side of the victim. Both of these forces deform the patient's body and create cavitation on the lateral aspect. When the patient is examined later in the emergency room, the depth and size of the deformation can be determined only by knowledge of the direction and force of the impact and a description of the passenger compartment intrusion. As will be described, three areas of the body are vulnerable to injury, two of which can involve the retroperitoneum.

One impact area that effects the retroperitoneum is the lateral trochanter. The head of the femur is pushed through the acetabulum into the retroperitoneum. Secondly, the wing of the ileum can be hit, fracturing the pelvis either at the sacral-iliac joint and symphysis pubis or fragmenting the bone in several pieces. The vascularity of the sacrum and muscles in the retroperitoneal area can produce extensive hemorrhage. Although there is no specific organ injury, this amount of blood loss can significantly affect patient survival. A full urinary bladder may rupture with external compression, and fractures of the pelvic bones may tear the urethra. The impact and subsequent cavitation of the lower rib cage on the lateral abdominal wall injure the intra-abdominal organs (spleen, driver side impact; and liver, passenger side impact). The rapid change in direction induces shear injuries to the kidney.

Vascular Shear Injuries

That portion of the aorta that is tightly tethered to the vertebral column by its fibrous attachments slows much more rapidly than the more freely movable organs such as the kidneys. The differential motion between these two components results in energy exchange that affects the vascular pedicle of the kidney. An analogy would be a golf ball tied to a rubber band and dropped. As long as the rubber band is stretching, the ball will continue to drop. If the elasticity of the rubber band is strong enough, the golf ball will eventually stop and return to its original position. However, if the elasticity of the rubber band is exceeded, the ball will be separated from the band and continue to fall. The golf ball in the analogy represents the kidney and the rubber band, the vascular pedicle. There can be three results of such decelerations: (1) the vascular pedicle is torn free, depriving the kidney of blood flow; (2) the pedicle is stretched so that the adventitia remains intact, but the intima is torn, clots forming at the turbulent area can occlude the vessel, the adventitia may stretch and form a pseudoaneurysm, or the adventitia may rupture, producing free hemorrhage into the retroperitoneal space; or (3) the vessel is not injured, the kidney has returned to its normal position, and its blood flow is not interrupted.

Pancreas

Blunt Injury

The pancreas' unique location, its adherence to the posterior abdominal wall, and its lack of a vascular pedicle—all reduce its susceptibility to shear injury but increase the probability of compressive injury. In a frontal impact when there is continued motion of the unrestrained occupant in a forward direction against the reduced motion of the vehicle, impacts of the anterior abdominal wall against the steering column or dashboard (or upper abdominal compression against an incorrectly applied lap restraint) rapidly stops the motion of the anterior abdominal wall. Continued motion of the vertebral column from behind compresses the center portion of the pancreas while allowing the head and tail to sink into areas of less rigidity (vertebral muscles) and the concavity of the gutters. The resultant forces will contuse or fracture the pancreas. Although the splenic artery and vein lie on the posterior surface of the pancreas in this area, they are not as easily injured.

Penetrating Injury

The significance of penetrating injury to organs is directly related to the energy exchange and therefore the size of the cavitation. Ischemic injury to the pancreatic tissue and duct, allowing delayed pancreatic enzyme rupture or accumulation of necrotic tissue to serve as a culture for bacterial growth and subsequent abscess formation, must be taken into consideration when accomplishing debridement.

Kidney

The location, lack of support, and pedicle of the kidney make it vulnerable to both compressive and deceleration (shear) forces in blunt trauma and cavitation in penetrating trauma.

As the anterior abdominal wall stops its forward motion against the steering column, dashboard, or seat belt, the continued motion of the posterior abdominal wall compresses the kidney against the posterior aspect of the anterior abdominal wall. The kidney parenchyma is contained within a fibrous capsule that tends to contain the compressive force. There are two possible results: (1) capillary and vascular rupture produces a hematoma inside the kidney that may expand until ischemia develops in the surrounding tissue (closed space mass effect); or (2) if the capsule ruptures, hemostases by compression is lost and major blood loss occurs. Containing the hematoma within the capsule acts as an early survival technique, since massive hemorrhage is controlled. However, since the energy is directed to within, affecting the parenchyma before the energy force escapes to the outside, more extensive damage is done to the renal tissue than if there were no capsule present. For minor injury, this effect is beneficial. For major energy exchange, it is detrimental.

The obvious diagnostic result is hematuria in the absence of extravasation of urine. This can induce a minor diagnostic dilemma, since minimal damage will cause hematuria. It therefore becomes difficult to distinguish between hematuria of major significance and that of minor significance (Chapter 12).

Penetrating trauma to the kidney tends to dissipate the energy to the inside without allowing the following compression waves to escape. An analogy would be to throw a rock into a pond. The waves produced by the rock spread out over the entire area of the pond. Dropping the same rock from the same high height into a bucket will force the waves to rebound back toward the center when the wave hits the wall of the container. The water particles inside the bucket are affected many times by back and forth wave motion, whereas there would be only one impact to the water particles in the large pond. Therefore, kidneys tend to shatter with direct penetrating trauma, demonstrating extensive fracture patterns within the capsule. Tissue destruction is massive and hemorrhage tends to be brisk.

SUMMARY

An understanding of some basic concepts of physics will allow an individual to comprehend injury patterns in both blunt and penetrating trauma. Examination of vehicle deformity will allow an estimation of the energy transferred to the victim. Injury patterns can be anticipated, depending on the force vectors imparted to the patient.

REFERENCES

1. Scalea T, Goldstein A, Phillips T, Sclafano SJA, Panetta T, McAuley J, Shaftan G: An analysis of 161 falls from a height: The 'jumper syndrome'. *J Trauma* 1986;26:706–712.
2. Fackler ML: Physics of missile injuries. In McSwain NE Jr, Kerstein MD (eds): *Evaluation and Management of Trauma*. Norwalk, CT: Appleton-Century-Crofts, 1987, pp. 25–41.
3. McSwain NE Jr: Abdominal trauma. In McSwain NE Jr, Kerstein MD (eds): *Evaluation and Management of Trauma*. Norwalk, CT: Appleton-Century-Crofts, 1987, pp. 129–167.
4. McSwain NE Jr: Mechanisms of injuries in blunt trauma. In McSwain NE Jr, Kerstein MD (eds): *Evaluation and Management of Trauma*. Norwalk, CT: Appleton-Century-Crofts, 1987, pp 1–24.
5. Fackler ML, Dougherty PJ: Theodor Kocher and the scientific foundation of wound ballistics. *Surg Gynecol Obstet* 1991;172:153–160.
6. Fackler ML, Malinowski JA: Internal deformation of the AK-74; a possible cause for its erratic path in tissue. *J Trauma* 1988;28(Suppl):S72–S75.
7. Walker ML, Poindexter JM Jr, Stovall I: Principles of management of shotgun wounds. *Surg Gynecol Obstet* 1990;170:97–105.
8. Ordog GJ, Wasserberger J, Balasubramaniam S: Shotgun wound ballistics. *J Trauma* 1988;28:624–631.
9. Grimes WR, Deitch E, McDonald JC: A clinical review of shotgun wounds to the chest and abdomen. *Surg Gynecol Obstet* 1985;160:148–152.
10. DeMuth WE Jr: Bullet velocity and design as determinants of wounding capability: An experimental study. *J Trauma* 1966;6:222–232.
11. Sykes LN Jr, Champion HR, Fouty WJ: Dum-dums, hollow-points, and devastators: Techniques designed to increase wounding potential of bullets. *J Trauma* 1988;28:618–623.

3

Initial Evaluation

SCOTT B. FRAME, M.D., F.A.C.S.

Retroperitoneal injuries often coexist with injuries to structures contained within the peritoneal cavity. Any trauma patient who arrives for care must be approached in a systematic manner so that all injuries are identified in the most expeditious fashion. Also, injuries may be present that pose an immediate threat to life, and these must be rapidly found and addressed. For these reasons, the initial evaluation and resuscitation does not differ from one trauma patient to the next. Only when associated injuries have been ruled out and the surgeon still has a high level of suspicion that a retroperitoneal injury is present do special studies related only to the retroperitoneal organs come into diagnostic prominence.

INITIAL EVALUATION AND RESUSCITATION

The basic approach to the victim of trauma holds for all patients who present for care. The consequences of trauma are often visually spectacular. The surgeon must not fall into the trap of being drawn to the most obvious external injuries, which usually do not pose an immediate threat to life, and ignore the less obvious injuries that may kill within seconds or minutes.

A sound, rational approach to the trauma patient has been outlined by the American College of Surgeons Committee on Trauma in the Advanced Trauma Life Support Course.[1] The first step in the care of any trauma patient is to ensure the patency of the airway and the adequacy of breathing. All trauma patients should be placed on supplemental oxygen, with high flow through a face mask being the preferred method of delivery. Nasal prongs will be mentioned only to condemn their use as being wholly inadequate as a source for supplemental oxygen for the trauma patient.

The next priority in caring for the injured patient is to reestablish adequate circulation. This calls for the placement of two large-bore intravenous lines. Large bore lines mean at least a 16 gauge, with 14 gauge catheters preferable. Central lines are not to be used as initial resuscitation lines, but are used for monitoring purposes only in the trauma patient. The antecubital fossa in the upper extremities is the primary site for intravenous access. In patients with injuries below the diaphragm, upper extremity access should be obtained to prevent the loss of resuscitation fluids into the injured abdominal cavity.

Another important aspect of the establishment and maintenance of normal perfusion is to stop ongoing blood loss. During the initial assessment and resuscitation phase, this includes control of obvious, external bleeding. This should be easily accomplished with direct pressure to the bleeding sites. Ongoing internal blood loss will need to be addressed in the operating room.

The fourth and fifth items to be performed in the initial evaluation are determination of neurologic disability and complete exposure of the patient so that all injuries may be identified. The neurologic examination, which is performed at this point, is abbreviated and should follow the AVPU format (A, alert; V, responds to verbal stimuli; P, responds to painful stimuli; or U, unresponsive). Exposure entails the removal of all clothing. Injuries that cannot be visualized will be missed with potentially disastrous results.

During the initial assessment, any immediately life-threatening injuries that are identified are addressed as they arise. These injuries include airway obstruction, tension pneumothorax, open pneumothorax, massive hemothorax, cardiac tamponade, and flail chest.

Gastric decompression and monitoring of urinary output is accomplished as soon as is conveniently feasible during the initial evaluation and resuscitation phases. Gastric decompression should be done via a nasogastric tube unless massive facial trauma is present, in which case an orogastric tube should be used. A Foley catheter is placed in the male only after the possibility of urethral disruption has been investigated. A transurethral tube is contraindicated in the presence of blood at the meatus, scrotal hematoma, or nonpalpable or high-riding prostate on rectal examination.

After the completion of the initial survey, the secondary survey is performed. It must be kept in mind that not all patients are stable enough to allow progression to the secondary survey. Some patients may never pass through the initial survey stage, but proceed directly to the operating room for surgical repair of life-threatening injuries. The life-threatening injuries are addressed as they are identified, so some patients may have injuries that preclude even the completion of the initial survey.

The secondary survey is a more detailed head-to-toe examination of the patient to identify all injuries and prioritize definitive treatment. This examination is also referred to as "fingers and tubes in every orifice." An uncommon finding during the secondary survey that may indicate a retroperitoneal injury is the presence of the Grey Turner sign. This sign is classically described in association with pancreatitis, but may be present as a retroperitoneal hematoma dissects into the flank. However, it is impossible to differentiate a flank contusion from dissected blood from a retroperitoneal hematoma.

GENERAL DIAGNOSTIC PROCEDURES

Not all patients require special and complicated diagnostic procedures. Valuable information may be obtained from the standard and simple tests that are routinely performed. Some tests should be obtained on all trauma patients and others are tailored to the particular needs of the patient.

The most common tests that are performed are obtained from the peripheral blood. It is standard procedure to draw the "Rainbow" pack of blood tubes on arrival of the patient in the emergency room. These laboratory studies include: (1) Complete blood count with hematocrit, red blood cell count, white blood cell count, and platelet count; (2) serum electrolytes, including sodium, potassium, chloride, carbon dioxide, glucose, and blood urea nitrogen; (3) serum creatinine, amylase, and liver function tests; (4) blood coagulation studies; (5) serum drug screen and blood alcohol; and (6) determination of blood type and crossmatch. Arterial blood gas determination is performed to ascertain the adequacy of oxygenation and ventilation, and the acid-base status of the patient. In addition to the blood studies, urine should also be obtained for dipstick analysis, immediate microscopic urinalysis, and drug screen.

Of the studies just listed, only blood type and crossmatch, arterial blood gases, and urinalysis are of immediate importance. Blood must be rapidly typed for potential administration. Immediate interventions may be dictated by the results of the blood gases, and the adequacy of the resuscitation endeavors may be followed through the status of the patient's acidosis. The presence of blood in the urine is an important piece of diagnostic information and will lead to the performance of more specialized tests to be described later.

The remainder of the studies have no immediate usefulness in the management of the patient, but are useful for establishing baselines for following the patient long-term. The initial hematocrit will probably be normal even in the presence of massive blood loss. Serial hematocrits are useful because they will demonstrate a decreasing value and give indications of possible continued blood loss. An elevated white blood cell count may be indicative of stress, drug or alcohol use, hemorrhage, or splenic damage. This is a very nonspecific sign and is not usually helpful in the acute setting. Serum electrolytes are also not immediately helpful, but serve as baselines for future comparison. The coagulation studies may be initially abnormal without clinical signs of a coagulopathy.[2] The significance of this finding has not been ascertained. The initial serum amylase appears to have little diagnostic value for pancreatic trauma.[3–5] However, serial determinations that demonstrate persistent elevation or a rising value may be helpful in indicating pancreatic damage.

Certain radiographs should be routinely obtained in every trauma patient. In the blunt trauma patient the chest radiograph, lateral cervical spine, and anteroposterior pelvic films are essential for the adequate evaluation of the patient. The pelvic film is necessary to rule out occult fractures that may not be demonstrated on physical examination.[6] In the patient with penetrating trauma, the chest radiograph should still be obtained and other films are obtained as they are clinically indicated. If an abdominal wound is present, anteroposterior and lateral abdominal films should be obtained after marking the entrance and exit wounds with radiopaque markers.

The value of plain abdominal films is in the detection of intra- or retroperitoneal fluid. The signs of intra-abdominal fluid include the flank strip sign, separation of the ascending and descending colon from the adjacent properitoneal fat; loss of definition of the hepatic angle (the hepatic angle sign); and the presence of homogenous shadows of water density in and adjacent to the pouch of Douglas (the "dog ear" sign).[4] Retroperitoneal hemorrhage may be indicated by abnormalities of the renal shadows or unilateral absence of the psoas shadow. The presence of a pelvic fracture also means that a retroperitoneal hematoma is present. The plain films may occasionally demonstrate air in the retroperitoneal space from perforation of a retroperitoneal hollow viscus, most commonly the duodenum (Fig. 3–1).

Diagnostic peritoneal lavage (DPL) remains the standard for the detection of intra-abdominal trauma, particularly in the blunt trauma patient. The use of DPL in the evaluation of penetrating abdominal trauma is less clear and the standards for considering a lavage positive varies from author to author. It must still be considered standard of care to explore the abdomens in all patients with gunshot wounds and all stab wounds that have been proven

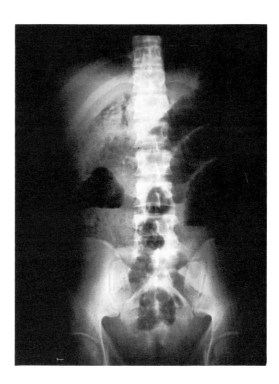

Figure 3–1. Abdominal radiograph demonstrating retroperitoneal air secondary to ruptured duodenum from blunt trauma.

by local exploration to penetrate the anterior rectus sheath. Exploration is to be especially encouraged in smaller hospitals where trauma is not routinely encountered. Further evaluation of DPL in the diagnosis of penetrating trauma should be reserved for the major trauma centers actively involved in research evaluation of the technique.

DPL has been shown to be inaccurate in the diagnosis of injuries isolated to the retroperitoneum.[7–9] The posterior parietal peritoneum isolates the extravasated blood from the peritoneal cavity and therefore the diagnostic "eyes" of DPL. Severe injuries may be present and the DPL will be negative. Most false-negative results of DPL can be attributed to missed retroperitoneal injuries. Since the mainstay of diagnosis for abdominal trauma is not effective, other means must be relied on when mechanism of injury indicates the possibility of retroperitoneal trauma.

Computed tomography (CT) is gaining support as a reliable means for evaluating the trauma patient in general, and the patient suspected of having isolated retroperitoneal trauma in particular. This study is the topic of Chapter 4 and will not be dealt with in depth at this time.

SPECIAL STUDIES

It must be kept in mind that the following special studies are reserved for those patients who are hemodynamically stable and have no strict indication for exploratory celiotomy. Time should not be wasted in obtaining needless tests when the decision has already been made to explore the patient. Once that decision has been made, the patient should be taken to the operating room with as little delay as possible. Remember, any patient may rapidly deteriorate no matter how "well" they may look.

Contrast Studies

Orally administered contrast medium is at times useful in diagnosing injuries to the upper gastrointestinal tract. The utility of these studies is extremely limited in the acute setting but in the stable patient may prove to be helpful. Extravasation of the contrast material from the duodenum either into the free peritoneal cavity or into the retroperitoneal space is diagnostic for duodenal perforation. Since extravasation of barium is to be avoided due to the extensive inflammatory reaction it incites, it is recommended that a water-soluble contrast medium be administered first. Blunt trauma may also result in an intramural hematoma of the duodenum. Once a laceration has been ruled out with water-soluble contrast medium, then barium may be given to provide better anatomic delineation of the duodenum. This is the diagnostic test of choice for duodenal hematoma. The pathognomonic findings are widened mucosal folds producing a characteristic pattern variously described as "accordion pleating," "picket fence," or "coiled spring" appearance. Extensive intramural hematoma may result in complete occlusion of the lumen with duodenal obstruction.[10]

Blunt trauma rarely causes damage to the colon, but sacrococcygeal fractures and extensive buttocks lacerations may result in rectal injuries. Penetrating injuries cause rectal trauma more frequently. When the rectal examination (required in *every* trauma patient) reveals the presence of blood, a rectal injury must be suspected and ruled out. The preferred method of diagnosis for rectal injuries is a proctoscopic examination with direct visualization of the defect. In the equivocal patient who remains stable, a water-soluble contrast enema may aid in the localization of a rectal laceration. In the author's experience it is extremely rare to have to resort to contrast enemas for the diagnosis of rectal injuries.

The contrast examination of the urogenital system is the mainstay of diagnosis of injuries to this organ system. Excretory urography or the intravenous pyelogram (IVP) is the most commonly utilized technique for the diagnosis of injuries to the kidneys or ureters.

In blunt trauma the indication for the performance of an IVP has traditionally been the presence of microscopic hematuria. This has recently come under attack by some authors.[11] However, the authors believe that the overwhelming preponderance of evidence favors the routine use of IVP in the blunt trauma patient when microscopic hematuria is present. The test has a low incidence of complications, the most common being allergic reaction to the dye. The consequence of a missed renal injury is possible loss of the kidney. When this is weighed against the small chance of complication, the scales definitely tip in favor of obtaining the IVP.

The indications for obtaining an IVP in penetrating trauma are more clear and simple. The presence of an abdominal wound requiring exploration should lead to an IVP. It is extremely useful to know prior to the start of exploration that two functioning renal units are present. This makes the decisions surrounding a possible nephrectomy versus repair to be made with the knowledge that a functioning kidney is or is not present on the other side. The knowledge of the presence of renal extravasation is also necessary to enable the proper decisions to be carried out when confronting a retroperitoneal hematoma (Chapters 5 and 12).

The technique for the IVP depends on the status of the patient and the mechanism of injury. In the unstable blunt trauma patient and the victim of penetrating trauma, the "one-shot" IVP should be used. This technique calls for the injection of 2 cc/kg of renal contrast medium up to 100 cc. A flat plate of the abdomen is then obtained approximately 1 to 3 minutes after injection. A minimal amount of information is sought from this test prior to the abdominal exploration. The presence or absence of bilateral renal function or extravasation are the only pieces of information that this study yields. In the stable blunt trauma patient, a formal IVP with nephrotomography is obtained.

Recently, CT has been touted as the diagnostic test of choice for the renal system. Again, this will be dealt with in greater detail in Chapters 4 and 12. The caution must be made that CT scans require the presence of an experienced trauma radiologist for accurate interpretation of the test.

Ultrasonography

The use of ultrasound as a diagnostic aid in the trauma patient in this country has been very limited. However, the Germans have expressed great confidence in the procedure and by verbal discussions at conferences it appears they use ultrasound in preference to CT scanning as a noninvasive diagnostic measure.

The reports from this country offer a somewhat different picture of the accuracy of ultrasound. In the diagnosis of splenic injury there have been reports of difficulty differentiating hematoma from the underlying splenic parenchyma.[12,13] In the evaluation of renal trauma ultrasound may provide anatomic data, but no information as to renal function. Ultrasonography can demonstrate the extent of perirenal hematoma, but cannot delineate parenchymal damage to any great extent.

The biggest problem with the use of ultrasonography in trauma is the difficulty in obtaining a technically adequate study. Bowel gas blocks the passage of the ultrasonic waves, which means that any organs lying beneath loops of gas-filled bowel cannot be visualized. Trauma patients often have an accompanying ileus, which obliterates the underlying structures. The most difficult structures to delineate are those in the retro-peritoneum, rendering this modality of limited benefit in the diagnosis of retroperitoneal trauma. Another limitation of the technique is that multiple scans in various positions must be performed in order to evaluate abdominal structures adequately. This is obviously difficult in the multitrauma patient. The presence of bandages and open wounds also limit the areas of the body that can be examined by ultrasound.

Radionuclide Scanning

During the acute phase of trauma, the use of radionuclide scanning is limited. The only scans used in the trauma setting with any regularity are the liver-spleen and renal scans. The use of radionuclide scanning in the diagnosis of diaphragmatic injury has recently been advocated.[14,15]

Liver-spleen scans may be useful in identifying larger parenchymal defects of these organs. Defects within the parenchyma may be seen as "cold" areas of nonfunctional parenchyma with surrounding compression of normal tissue. Indications of perihepatic or perisplenic hematomas may be found on scanning when the lateral contour of the organ is flattened and the lateral abdominal wall is displaced.[16–18] These findings are subtle and may be easily overlooked. False-positive results may be secondary to congenital clefts, cysts, tumors, or infarctions.

Renal scans may be used to ascertain renal function in the stable patient with nonvisualization of a kidney on IVP. Delayed images may reveal large parenchymal defects, but the resolution is poor and small injuries may be easily missed. The most important information obtained is on renal function and vascular integrity of the renal units.

Arteriography

The use of arteriography as a diagnostic and therapeutic modality in both blunt and penetrating trauma has grown steadily over the last several years. In the past arteriograms have been mainly recommended as a follow-up study in those patients who have nondiagnostic plain films or radionuclide scans.

Renal arteriography is recommended when there is a nonfunctional kidney, evidence of major parenchymal damage, or equivocal study on IVP. The arteriogram may or may not be preceded by renal radionuclide scanning. Renal arteriography is able to identify accurately parenchymal injuries and differentiate contusions and small cortical lacerations; renal pedicle injuries are best delineated by the study.

The diagnosis of injuries to the liver and spleen may also be made via arteriography, although other, less invasive studies are preferable for this purpose. Abdominal arteriography may demonstrate extravasation of contrast into parenchymal fractures, early venous filling, displacement of normal vascular architecture by hematoma, and nonhomogeneous enhancement of the organ during the capillary phase.[19,20] False-positive results may be caused by congenital abnormalities.

Arteriography may also demonstrate arteriovenous fistulas, false aneurysms, and arteriobiliary fistulas. These conditions are usually found in penetrating trauma.

The value of arteriography in the therapeutic arena lies in the ability to embolize bleeding vessels. Hemorrhage from pelvic fractures is especially suited to embolization, as outlined in Chapter 13. Lumbar artery embolization has also been described.[21]

The role of embolization in the treatment of renal injuries is much less important. Most renal injuries do well with conservative therapy and do not come to either surgical repair or embolization. Renal injuries resulting in hypotension in the acute phase are treated via surgical intervention. The role of arteriography lies in the treatment of those injuries resulting in persistent or repeated hematuria; slow, steady blood loss requiring transfusion; and significant defects, found while performing arteriography, that may cause complications in the future. These include large arteriovenous fistulas and pseudoaneurysms. Such indications rarely arise.[21]

The major limitation of arteriography lies in the selectivity of the test. To obtain technically adequate studies that allow accurate diagnosis, selective vessel cannulation must be performed. To "search" the abdomen for injuries would require multiple vessel cannulation with large dye loads. This greatly extends the time required to perform the procedure and increases the morbidity and mortality of the study.

Endoscopy

Both endoscopic gastroduodenoscopy (EGD) and colonoscopy have very little use in the acutely injured patient. Most indications for these procedures lie in the late phases of patient care when the long-term complications begin to manifest themselves. EGD itself should not be performed in the acute phase if perforation is suspected because the large volumes of air injected during the performance of the study may worsen the patient's situation. Colonoscopy in the unprepared colon is not only difficult to perform but is riskier due to lack of good visualization during the procedure. Also, diagnosis of subtle conditions is essentially impossible in the unprepared bowel.

Endoscopic Retrograde Cholangiopancreatography

Recent reports[22,23] have described the use of endoscopic retrograde cholangiopancreatography (ERCP) for the diagnosis of isolated pancreatic injuries secondary to trauma. The study can be performed in most patients and offers excellent visualization of the pancreatic duct. This allows identification of pancreatic duct disruption due to trauma, both blunt and penetrating.

SUMMARY

The most common means of diagnosing retroperitoneal trauma is via exploratory celiotomy for associated intra-abdominal injuries. A retroperitoneal hematoma is found and the injured organ thereby identified. For this type of patient, diagnostic peritoneal lavage is an excellent test. However, in the patient with isolated injuries in the retroperitoneum, DPL has a high rate of false-negative results, rendering it useless as an immediate diagnostic test. When isolated retroperitoneal trauma is suspected by mechanism of injury and clinical presentation, other modalities must be relied on to aid the physician in establishing a diagnosis.

Routinely obtained tests may give indications of the presence of injury. Plain radiographs of the abdomen, chest, and pelvis in the blunt trauma patient may give valuable clues or show pathognomonic signs. Contrast studies, especially the IVP, are extremely useful in some patients. CT is gaining support as the diagnostic test of choice for the retroperitoneum and is the subject of the next chapter. Special studies including ultrasonography, radionuclide scanning, arteriography, endoscopy, and ERCP all may be of diagnostic and therapeutic benefit in selected patients. All of the special studies are reserved for those patients who are hemodynamically stable.

REFERENCES

1. American College of Surgeons Committee on Trauma: Abdominal Trauma. In *Advanced Trauma Life Support Course, Student Manual*. Chicago: American College of Surgeons, 1988, pp 111–125.
2. Timberlake GA, McSwain NE: Coagulopathy in hypotensive trauma patients: A laboratory finding in search of significance. First Annual Scientific Meeting of the *Eastern Association for the Surgery of Trauma*; Longboat Key, Florida. (Abstr.) January 15, 1988.

3. Olsen WR: The serum amylase in blunt abdominal trauma. *J Trauma* 1973;13:200–204.
4. Trunkey DD, Federle MP, Cello JP: Special diagnostic procedures. In Blaisdell FW, Trunkey DD (eds): *Abdominal Trauma*. New York: Thieme-Stratton, 1982, pp 19–43.
5. Weigelt JA: Duodenal injuries. *Surg Clin North Am* 1990;70:529–539.
6. Gillot A, Rhodes M, Leuke J, et al: Utility of routine pelvic x-ray in blunt trauma resuscitation. *J Trauma* 1988;28:1570–1574.
7. Hubbard SG, Bivens BA, Sachatello CR, et al: Diagnostic errors with peritoneal lavage in patients with pelvic fractures. *Arch Surg* 1979;114:844–846.
8. Parvin S, Smith DG, Asher M, et al: Effectiveness of diagnostic peritoneal lavage in blunt trauma. *Ann Surg* 1975;181:255–261.
9. Cogbill TH, Moore EE, Feliciano DV, et al: Conservative management of duodenal trauma: A multicenter perspective. *J Trauma* 1990;30:1469–1475.
10. Mahboubi S, Kaufmann HJ: Intramural duodenal hematoma in children: The role of the radiologist in its conservative management. *Gastrointest Radiol* 1976;1:167–171.
11. Klein S, Johs S, Fujitani R, et al: Hematuria following blunt abdominal trauma—the utility of intravenous pyelography. *Arch Surg* 1988;123:1173–1177.
12. Wilson RL, Rogers WF, Shaub MS: Splenic subcapsular hematoma—ultrasonic diagnosis. *West J Med* 1978; 128:6–8.
13. Asher WM, Parvin S, Virgilio RW, et al: Echographic evaluation of splenic injury after blunt trauma. *Radiology* 1976;118:411–415.
14. Kim EE, McConnell BJ, McConnell RW, et al: Radionuclide diagnosis of diaphragmatic rupture with herniation. *Surgery* 1983;94:36–40.
15. Pecoraro JP, Shea LM, Tenorio LE, et al: Radioisotope-assisted diagnosis of traumatic rupture of the diaphragm. *Am Surg* 1985;51:687–689.
16. Nesbesar RA, Rabinov KR, Potsaid MS: Radionuclide imaging of the spleen in suspected splenic injury. *Radiology* 1974;110:609–614.
17. Lutzker L, Koenigsberg M, Meng CH, et al: The role of radionuclide imaging in splenic trauma. *Radiology* 1974;110:419–425.
18. Evans GW, Curtin G, McCarthy HF, et al: Scintigraphy in traumatic lesions of the liver and spleen. *JAMA* 1972;222:665–667.
19. Redman HC, Reuter SR, Bookstein JJ: Angiography in abdominal trauma. *Ann Surg* 1969;169:57–66.
20. Berk RW, Wholey MH, Stackdale RL: The angiographic diagnosis of splenic and hepatic trauma. *J Can Assoc Radiol* 1970;21:230–234.
21. Sclafani SJA, Becker JA: Interventional radiology in the treatment of retroperitoneal trauma. *Urol Radiol* 1985;7:219–230.
22. Hayward SR, Lucas CE, Sugawa C, et al: Emergent endoscopic retrograde cholangiopancreatography; a highly specific test for acute pancreatic trauma. *Arch Surg* 1989;124:745–746.
23. Whittwell AE, Gomez GA, Byers P, et al: Blunt pancreatic trauma: Prospective evaluation of early endoscopic retrograde pancreatography. *South Med J* 1989;82:586–591.

4

Computed Tomography in Retroperitoneal Trauma

KIMBALL I. MAULL, M.D., F.A.C.S.
HOWARD R. GOULD, M.D.

Injuries to structures lying in the retroperitoneal space present several hazards to the patient and to the unwary physician responsible for the patient's care. Of most immediate concern is exsanguination from vascular damage, which challenges the technical expertise of the surgeon. Of equal concern is missed injury, which challenges the physician as diagnostician. It is clear that there may be few or no clinical signs or symptoms at a time when significant, even life-threatening, retroperitoneal injuries exist. For these reasons, diagnostic aids beyond clinical assessment are essential to assure timely diagnosis and, if needed, prompt operative intervention.

ROLE OF COMPUTED TOMOGRAPHY IN ABDOMINAL TRAUMA

In 1830, Hazlitt stated "when a subject ceases to be a matter of controversy, it ceases to be a subject of interest." In recent years, few topics have generated as much controversy or as much interest as defining the role of computed tomography (CT) in the diagnosis of abdominal trauma. Diagnostic peritoneal lavage (DPL), a safe and sensitive indicator of intraperitoneal bleeding, occupied center stage in the diagnostic armamentarium of the trauma surgeon since its original description by Root in 1965.[1] With a test that detects intra-abdominal injury reliably and rapidly, why stray from the chosen path? In 1985, the first reports comparing CT and DPL were published.[2,3] Additional studies have appeared in the literature since 1985.[4-6]

It is not the intent of this chapter to debate this issue. Both CT and DPL are accurate and reliable in detecting intra-abdominal injury. Both techniques have pitfalls.[7,8] Yet, even the most ardent proponent of DPL would admit that lavage is of little value in detecting retroperitoneal injury unless there is concurrent intraperitoneal injury leading to operation. It is the role of CT in the diagnosis of retroperitoneal injuries that will remain the focus for this chapter.

PREREQUISITES FOR A SAFE COMPUTED TOMOGRAPHY EVALUATION

Except for a small number of newly designed trauma units in which the CT scanner is present in the resuscitation area, patients who require CT must be transported from the emergency unit to the radiology department to be studied. Therefore the patient *must be stable*.[9,10] It is important to remember that stability implies a steady state over time. An isolated recording of a normal blood pressure does not define stability and complete clinical assessment of the patient must be done first in order to determine the safety of obtaining a CT scan. The patient must be attended by qualified personnel who can monitor changes in the patient's condition, recognize meaningful trends, and institute appropriate remedial actions, if necessary. This means a physician and nurse team for, despite the best efforts at excluding unstable patients, any acutely injured patient may suddenly deteriorate and immediate therapeutic decisions are sometimes necessary. This problem is not confined to CT for abdominal trauma, but may also be seen in the head-injured patient who has concurrent but unsuspected torso injuries.

In order to obtain quality images, the patient must be still. Although many patients cooperate fully with verbal instructions, there are also many under the influence of drugs or alcohol who are uncooperative and require sedation or total paralysis. The latter is also true for young children in whom total control by intubation, ventilation, and muscle relaxants may occasionally be necessary. New, short exposure time scanners, such as 200 msec, may obviate this need.

INDICATIONS AND CONTRAINDICATIONS

Indications for CT and DPL are basically identical (Table 4–1). Any patient who presents at risk of abdominal injury with an unreliable examination should be considered for CT evaluation. There are additional specific indications for CT beyond its role as a screening tool. Repeat CT scanning may be indicated when an evolving process is suspected, if the

**Table 4–1 Indications for Computed Tomography
of the Abdomen in the Injured**

Indeterminate abdominal examinations
Head injury
Spinal injury
Drugs/alcohol
Associated chest wall injury
Hematuria
Pelvic fractures

initial scan was technically lacking, or to monitor (or drain) intra-abdominal or pelvic fluid collections.

CT is contraindicated in the unstable patient whether the patient is in the emergency unit or in an inpatient intensive care unit setting. In either instance, other diagnostic modalities, such as sonography, that do not require transport of the patient from the relative safety of the clinical setting should be considered.[11] Hypersensitivity to intravenous contrast is a relative contraindication insofar as an unenhanced CT affords less information and may confuse the clinician and radiologist alike.

TECHNICAL CONSIDERATIONS

The CT technique is critical in obtaining an optimal examination. All intravenous lines, electrodes, transducers, and enteric tubes should be out of the scanning field as much as possible. The lower chest and pelvis are included. A few images of the upper abdomen are obtained before giving intravenous contrast medium. These preliminary cuts have been helpful in defining hyperdense hematomas, which can be difficult to visualize following intravenous contrast medium administration. Active bleeding can be more apparent by comparing pre- and postcontrast scans (Fig. 4–1).

If a large, clinically unsuspected hemoperitoneum is discovered with the initial cuts, the patient may be taken immediately to the operating room without completing the contrast medium phase of the scan. Oral or rectal contrast medium may be helpful in diagnosing injuries to hollow viscera and is used on specific indication. However, oral contrast medium in particular can delay completion of the scan and is not used routinely.

Intravenous contrast medium appropriately delivered and sequenced with the images is a prerequisite for an adequate CT scan.[10] A bolus dynamic technique with power injection is used for the upper abdomen with rapid scanning inferiorly to the symphysis pubis. Lastly, we believe direct involvement by an experienced radiologist at the time of the scan is important. Diagnoses rendered the following day are of little help when rapid and often lifesaving decisions must be made in the middle of the night.

EVALUATION OF SPECIFIC ORGANS

Duodenum

The missed duodenal injury is one of the most dangerous retroperitoneal injuries. Duodenal injury occurs in approximately 5% of patients with blunt trauma to hollow viscera.[12] Gas outlining the right kidney on a plain abdominal film is considered pathognomonic, but the sign may be subtle or absent and abdominal films are not usually secured as part of the initial injured patient assessment.

Duodenal injuries should be suspected by mechanism of injury, when physical findings point toward upper abdominal trauma or whenever an elevated serum amylase level is identified.

Findings on CT may also be subtle. Thickening of the duodenal wall or extraluminal fluid about the duodenum or head of the pancreas are suggestive (Fig. 4–2). Contrast medium, either orally or per nasogastric tube, may resolve the issue (Figs. 4–3, 4–4). We

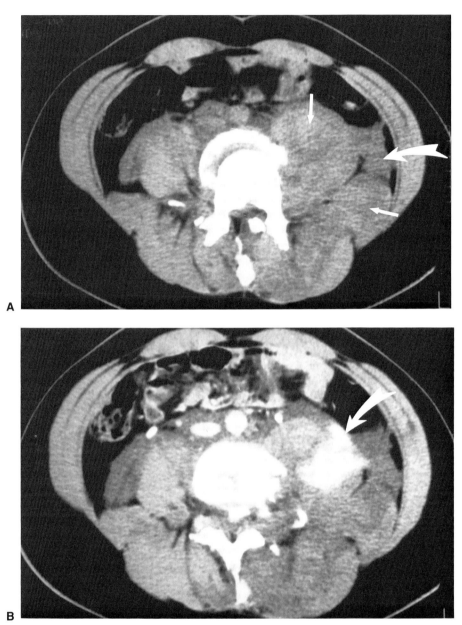

Figure 4–1. Active retroperitoneal hemorrhage with spinal fracture. **A:** Precontrast medium scan shows retroperitoneal hemorrhage (curved arrow) with enlarged psoas and quadratus (small arrows). **B:** Postcontrast medium scan shows active hemorrhage into left psoas (curved arrow).

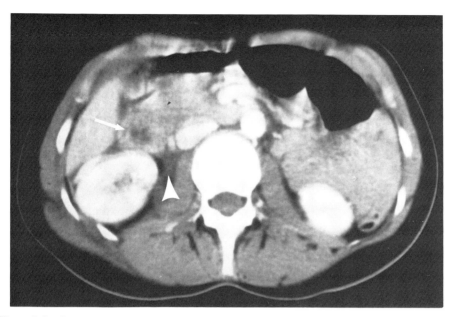

Figure 4–2. Ruptured duodenum. Scan without oral contrast medium shows thick-walled duodenum (arrow) and retroperitoneal fluid (arrowhead) adjacent to psoas.

favor standard water-soluble contrast medium for upper gastrointestinal series following CT if a duodenal injury is suspected, whereas others believe that CT with prior oral contrast medium is just as reliable.[13]

Pancreas

Injury to the pancreas demands prompt diagnosis and appropriate surgical therapy to avoid significant mortality or morbidity. Unfortunately, actual definition of the anatomy of injury may be obscured by hematoma and peripancreatic edema. Actual transection may be missed on initial scans only to be readily identifiable on later studies. In other instances, significant abnormalities are immediately discernible (Fig. 4–5). Nonetheless, combined with clinical and laboratory parameters, CT can be of considerable assistance in demonstrating injury to the pancreas and adjacent vital structures and lead to early operation (Figs. 4–6, 4–7). Thickening and infiltration of the left anterior renal fascia should raise suspicion of pancreatic injury.[14]

CT scanning is also valuable in following pancreatic injuries and complications resulting therefrom. This is particularly true relative to post-traumatic pancreatitis, pseudocyst and other consequences of ductal disruption and drainage.

Retroperitoneal Colon

Parts of the ascending and descending colon are retroperitoneal in location. Peritoneal signs may be masked by the retroperitoneal site of injury and delayed recognition may re-

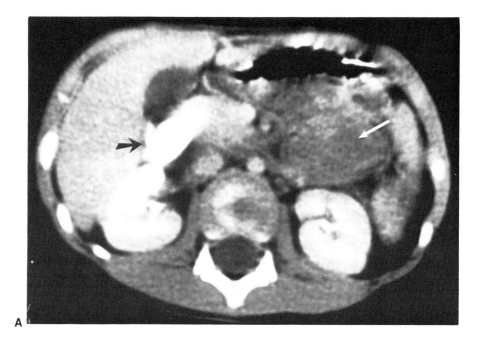

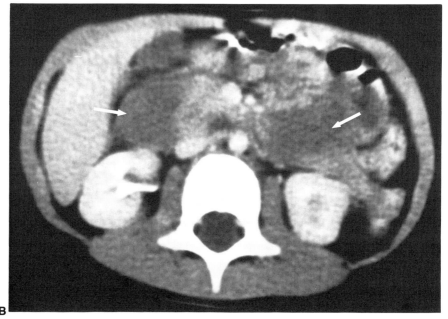

Figure 4–3.   Intramural hematoma of duodenum. A 3-year-old child suspected of being abused. **A:** Computed tomography scan showing contrast medium in proximal duodenum (black arrow) and hematoma (white arrow) in proximal jejunum. **B:** Next slice caudal to A showing hematoma (arrows) in the descending duodenum and in the fourth portion of the duodenum.

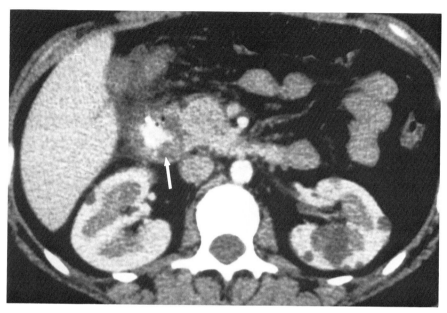

Figure 4–4. Intramural hematoma in the duodenum. Thick-walled duodenum (arrow) with irregular contrast-filled lumen. Minimal infiltration of the periduodenal fat but no extravasation.

sult in septic complications. Meyer et al[15] attest to the reliability of CT in stab wounds of the back. Although the authors did not employ rectal contrast medium, Phillips et al[16] cite CT enema as an important and accurate tool in defining penetrating colon injury. Blunt injury to the colon may also occur and appears to be increasing in frequency. In a recent report by Appleby and Nagy,[17] one third of hollow visceral injuries attributed to safety restraints were located in the colon.

Focal bowel wall thickening may indicate intramural hematoma. Focal pericolic infiltration and hemorrhage with or without extraluminal air are warning signs of colon injury. Whenever colon injury is suspected, confirmation by CT enema or standard water-soluble contrast medium enema examination is warranted. In our experience, retroperitoneal bowel injury is much less common than intraperitoneal injuries.

Genitourinary System

A normal excretory urogram excludes significant upper renal tract injury. However, an abnormal excretory urogram may not accurately stage the severity or type of injury and additional imaging studies with additional intravenous contrast are necessary. When CT is available, it is our belief that it is the preferred method of evaluation for possible renal injury. Devascularization, infarction, fracture, contusion, and extravasation are easily demonstrated by CT (Figs. 4–8, 4–9). Because of improved images and better definition of the anatomy of the injury, many patients undergoing exploration in the past are now being successfully managed nonoperatively.[18]

Using a bolus dynamic scanning technique alone will not provide adequate contrast

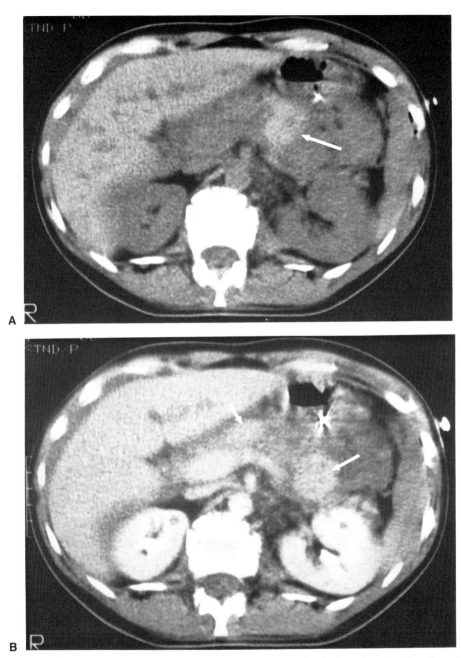

Figure 4–5.   Transection of the pancreas. **A:** Precontrast medium scan showing hyperdense hematoma (arrow) in pancreas. **B:** Postcontrast medium scan shows that this area does not enhance, whereas the remainder of pancreas does (arrows).

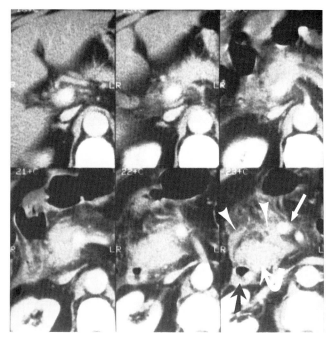

Figure 4–6. Peripancreatic hemorrhage. Multiple slices show peripancreatic hemorrhage (arrowheads) secondary to avulsion of uncinate vein from superior mesenteric vein (white arrow). Note duodenum (black arrow) and uncinate process (curved white arrow).

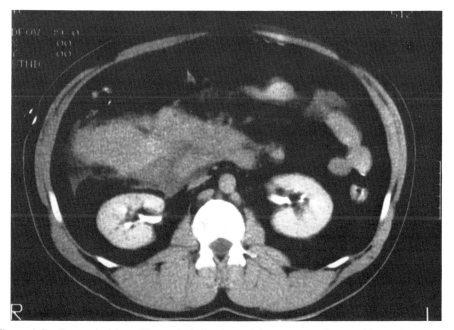

Figure 4–7. Pancreatic injury. Mesenteric infiltration and hematoma contiguous with anterior aspect of pancreatic head and duodenum secondary to a coronal transection of the pancreatic head.

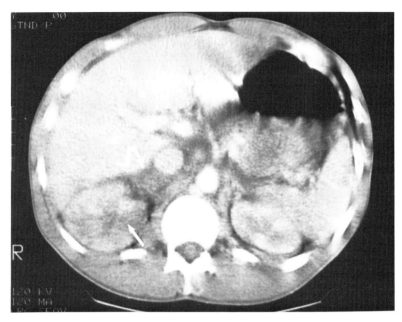

Figure 4–8.   Renal injury. Hemorrhage behind inferior vena cava (curved arrow) secondary to avulsion of the adrenal vein. Irregular fracture of right kidney (arrow). Other slices showed function with no extravasation.

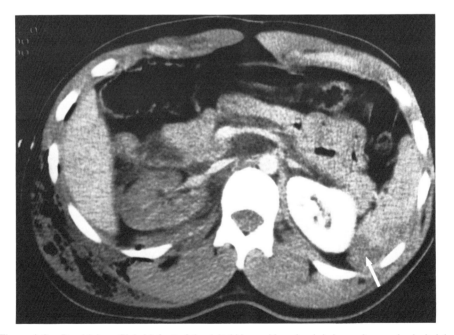

Figure 4–9.   Renal injury. Global infarct of the right kidney with perinephric hemorrhage and splenic injury (arrow). The left kidney enhances normally.

in the renal pelvis and ureter. We favor administering 5 ml of intravenous contrast medium a few minutes before the main injection. If there is not adequate contrast medium in the collecting systems and ureters, and if there is any fluid in the surrounding tissues, then delayed scans of the area are performed to exclude extravasation.

Early CT scanning can also identify the nonfunctioning kidney and presumed pedicle injury, leading to early arteriography and exploration. Unfortunately, most of these kidneys cannot be saved (Figs. 4–10, 4–11).

CT can identify ureteral injury by disclosing extravasation of contrast into the surrounding retroperitoneal soft tissue (Fig. 4–12). This injury, rare following blunt trauma, may be seen following penetrating wounds and is an injury to be excluded with flank and back stab wounds. Retrograde pyelography provides more definitive detail of the injury.

Contrast-enhanced CT may provide evidence of laceration to the urinary bladder (Fig. 4–13). The accumulation of contrast outside the confines of the bladder indicates bladder rupture (Fig. 4–14). Intraperitoneal and extraperitoneal rupture of the bladder can be differentiated by CT. Extraperitoneal rupture can be more subtle and difficult to diagnose. A negative CT examination does not exclude bladder injury and all patients with hematuria receive a standard retrograde cystogram.

Pelvic Fractures and Other Musculoskeletal Injuries

Pelvic fractures constitute a major problem in management of the acutely injured patient. Although pelvic fractures may be of little or no consequence when stable and undisplaced,

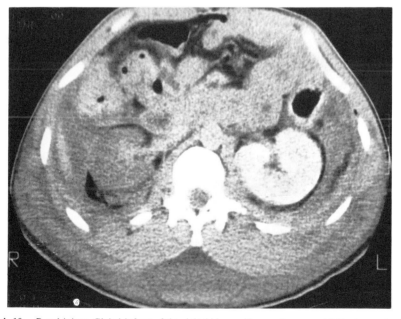

Figure 4–10. Renal injury. Global infarct of the right kidney with no enhancement following contrast.

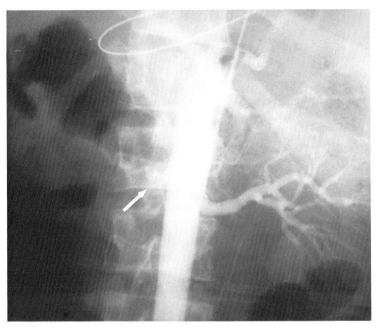

Figure 4–11.   Renal injury. Same patient as in Figure 10. Aortogram shows complete occlusion of the right renal artery (arrow).

unstable fractures may be rapidly fatal from associated intrapelvic retroperitoneal hemorrhage (Fig. 4–15). Paradoxically, the most severely injured (and often unstable) patient may require transport to the radiology suite for angiographic control of intrapelvic arterial bleeding. Nonetheless, CT scanning for pelvic injuries should adhere to the previous caveat requiring a stable patient.[19] Unlike angiography, CT scanning remains only a diagnostic modality in patients with suspected pelvic trauma.

The principal indications for CT in patients with pelvic fractures are to evaluate the genitourinary system, to define better the bony anatomy of the pelvis, and to assess for retroperitoneal hemorrhage. The anteroposterior (AP) pelvic film is routinely performed in all patients at risk, yet it is not a good screening study. Gross malalignment and bony disruption may be evident on the AP view but the more subtle findings of acetabular fractures and sacral fractures in particular are often underestimated or not apparent on the plain AP film. CT scan is a highly accurate technique for demonstrating the site and extent of pelvic injury, the size and distribution of pelvic hematoma, and may demonstrate injury to adjacent viscera.

Because CT scanning provides excellent structural definition, injuries may be discovered that were unsuspected by the clinician (Fig. 4–16). This certainly occurs with intraperitoneal injury, but it is also true for retroperitoneal trauma as well. Changes in bony relationships can implicate associated ligamentous tears and provide inferential data regarding stability and other structures at risk of injury (Fig. 4–17).

The retroperitoneal space has the capacity to hold a large amount of fluid. With CT, fluid can usually be easily identified, and in most cases categorized as to whether it is

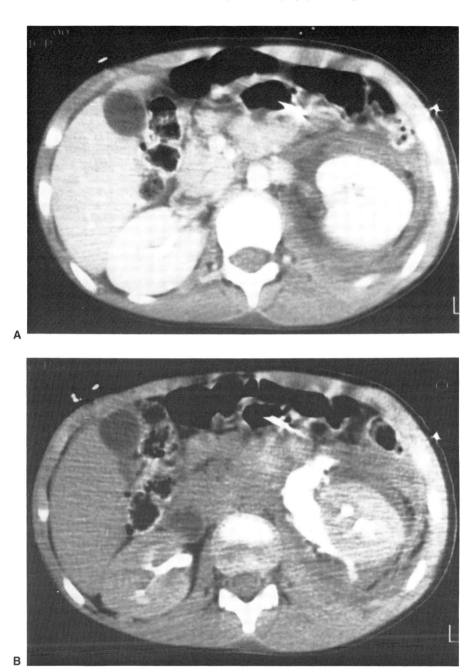

Figure 4–12. Avulsion of ureter from the renal pelvis. **A:** Initial scan shows normally enhancing kidney surrounded by fluid. **B:** Delayed scan with extensive extravasation of contrast.

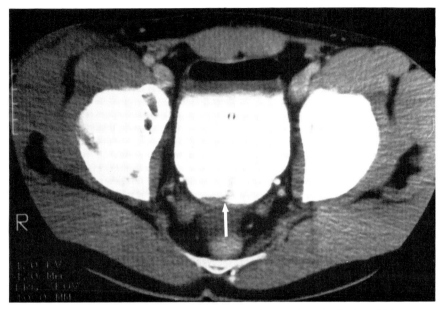

Figure 4–13. Bladder injury. Localized flap and tear (arrow) in posterior wall of urinary bladder.

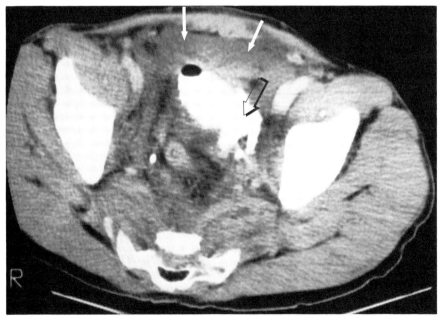

Figure 4–14. Bladder injury. Extraperitoneal bladder rupture with extraluminal contrast (open arrow) at the left lateral aspect of the bladder. Unopacified hemorrhage in the anterior extraperitoneal space (arrows).

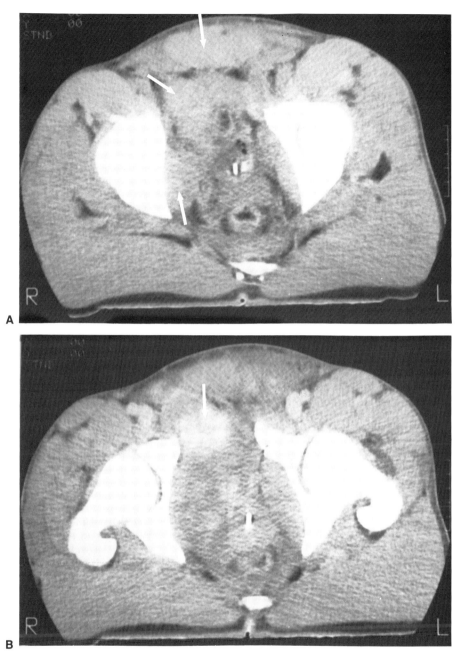

Figure 4–15. Pelvic fracture. **A:** Extensive extraperitoneal hemorrhage on precontrast scan (arrows). **B:** Leak of contrast (arrow) from bleeding vessels after contrast administration.

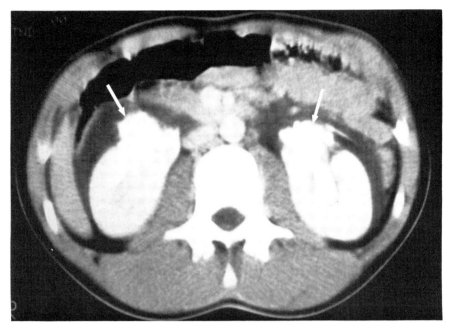

Figure 4–16. Urinary extravasation. Horseshoe kidney with bilateral urinomas and leak of contrast (arrows) from anteriorly located renal pelves.

blood or water density. Retroperitoneal hemorrhage from pelvic fractures can extend in the retroperitoneum to a point cephalic to the kidneys (Fig. 4–18). Although a source for the hemorrhage can usually be demonstrated, there are some cases in which it is never found. Nonhemorrhagic fluid can arise from retroperitoneal bowel injuries, lymphatic injuries, and "third spacing" (Figs. 4–19, 4–20).

Differentiation of intraperitoneal from extraperitoneal fluid is sometimes difficult, but is of critical importance, since intraperitoneal fluid or blood often indicates a need for celiotomy (Figs. 4–20, 4–21).

SURGICAL IMPLICATIONS OF CT FINDINGS

The retroperitoneal space has for decades been regarded as the "black box" of the abdomen. Because of its protected and relatively remote location, retroperitoneal disease processes may present late, resulting in delayed treatment and increased morbidity. The use of CT scanning in the acutely injured patient has suddenly opened this "black box" and provided early illumination of the region so treatment can be initiated promptly. Early recognition of duodenal and pancreatic injuries can improve outcome provided that surgical therapy follows without delay (Fig. 4–22). Ureteral repair before urinoma formation and closure of colonic wounds soon after injury may prevent the need for a second operation for reconstruction or stomal closure.

Although it is true that most retroperitoneal injuries do not occur in isolation, some do and these are the most dangerous.

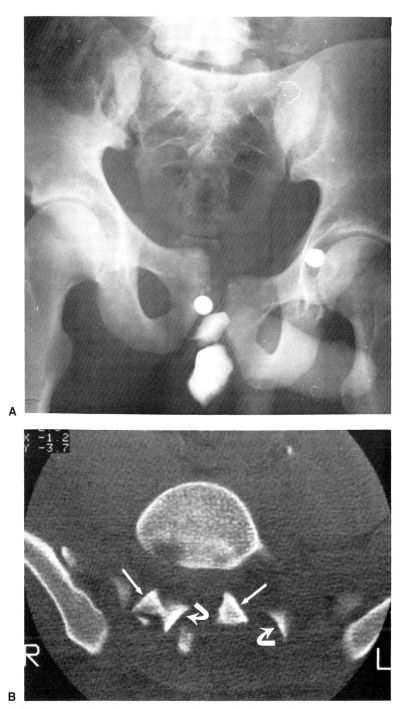

Figure 4–17.   Fracture of the pelvis. **A:** Fracture of the symphysis pubis, bilateral sacroiliac joint subluxation, and dislocation of L5-S1. **B:** Computed tomography scan showing lateral jumped facets of L5 and S1. Inferior facets L5 (arrows) and superior facets S1 (curved arrows).

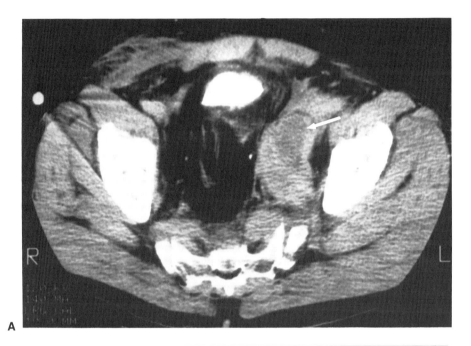

A

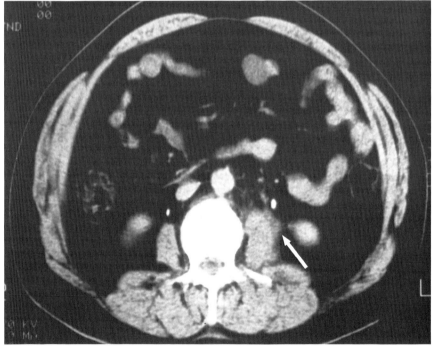

B

Figure 4–18.   Retroperitoneal hemorrhage. **A:** Pelvic fracture with extraperitoneal hemorrhage (arrow). **B:** Retroperitoneal extension of pelvic hematoma (arrow) extends to level of the left kidney.

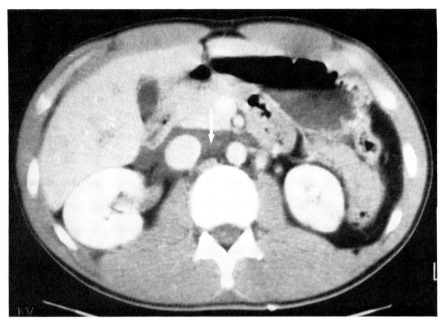

Figure 4–19. Ruptured cisterna chyli. Water density of the retroperitoneal fluid (arrow) was found to represent lymph from ruptured cisterna chyli.

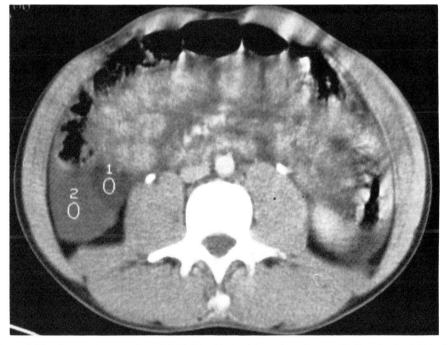

Figure 4–20. Intra- and extraperitoneal fluid. Blood in the right peritoneal gutter (2). Low-density fluid in the retroperitoneal space (1) secondary to "third spacing" in a patient with a ruptured spleen.

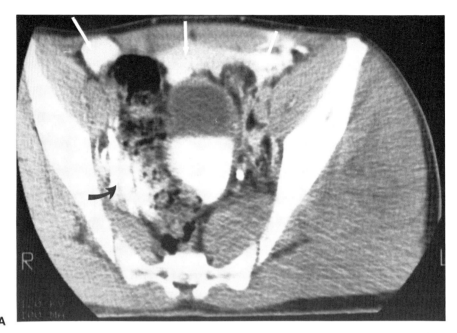

A

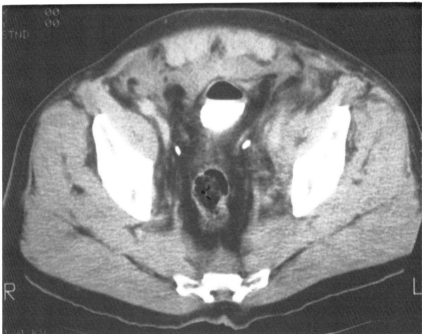

B

Figure 4–21. Extraperitoneal space. **A:** Extraperitoneal contrast (black and white arrows) following urethrogram for transection of membranous urethra. **B:** Another patient with extraperitoneal hemorrhage secondary to pelvic fracture. Note similarity of extraperitoneal space anteriorly and the absence of fluid in the cul-de-sac between the bladder and rectum.

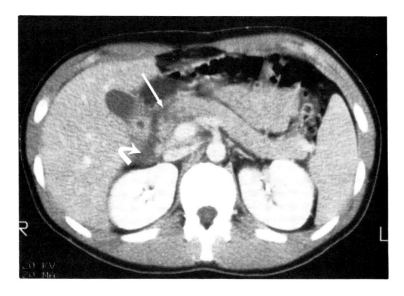

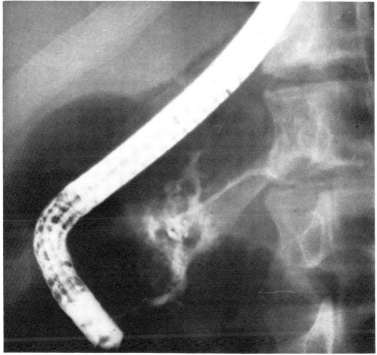

Figure 4–22. Pancreatic injury. **A:** Computed tomography scan showing cleft (arrow) at cephalic aspect of pancreatic head with some adjacent fluid (curved arrow) in a patient with minimal abdominal findings and hyperamylasemia. Endoscopic retrograde cholangiopancreatography (ERCP) recommended. **B:** ERCP shows extravasation from the ductal system. Operation followed promptly, confirming transection of the pancreatic duct.

CONCLUSIONS

Retroperitoneal injuries jeopardize the patient from exsanguination and from delay in recognition. CT scanning provides useful and timely information and is the diagnostic method of choice for the evaluation of retroperitoneal injuries. CT can provide precise anatomic detail and weigh heavily in the decision to operate or not operate, depending on the organ system involved and the defined extent of injury. CT may also be of benefit in following patients with known injuries and for detecting postinjury or postoperative retroperitoneal complications.

REFERENCES

1. Root HD, Hauser CW, McKinley CR, et al: Diagnostic peritoneal lavage. *Surgery* 1965;57:633–637.
2. Marx JA, Moore EE, Jorden RC, et al: Limitations of computed tomography in the evaluation of acute abdominal trauma: A prospective comparison with diagnostic peritoneal lavage. *J Trauma* 1985;25: 933–937.
3. Goldstein AS, Sclafani SJA, Kupperstein NH, et al: The diagnostic superiority of computerized tomography. *J Trauma* 1985;25:938–946.
4. Fabian TC, Mangiante EC, White TJ, et al: A prospective study of 91 patients undergoing both computed tomography and peritoneal lavage following blunt abdominal trauma. *J Trauma* 1986;26:602–608.
5. Meyer DM, Thal ER, Weigelt JA: Evaluation of computed tomography and diagnostic peritoneal lavage in blunt abdominal trauma. *J Trauma* 1989;29:1168–1172.
6. Frame SB, Browder IW, Lang EK, et al: Computed tomography versus diagnostic peritoneal lavage: Usefulness in immediate diagnosis of blunt abdominal trauma. *Ann Emerg Med* 1989;18:513–516.
7. Hornyak SW, Shaftan GW: Value of "inconclusive lavage" in abdominal trauma management. *J Trauma* 1979;19:329–332.
8. Gould HR, Buntain WL, Maull KI: Imaging in blunt abdominal trauma. *Adv Trauma* 1988;3:53–99.
9. Matsubara TK, Fong HMT, Burns CM: Computed tomography of abdomen (CTA) in management of blunt abdominal trauma. *J Trauma* 1990;30:410–414.
10. Jeffrey RB, Olcott EW: Imaging of blunt hepatic trauma. *Radiol Clin North Am* 1991;29:1299–1310.
11. Jones TK, Walsh JW, Maull KI: Diagnostic imaging in blunt trauma of the abdomen. *Surgery* 1983;157: 389–398.
12. Maull KI: Traumatic lesions of the duodenum. In HW Scott & JL Sawyers (eds.) *Surgery of the Stomach, Duodenum, and Small Intestine* Ed. 2. Boston: Blackwell Scientific Publications, 1992.
13. Sclafani SJA: Advances in trauma radiology. *Adv Trauma* 1986;1:71–84.
14. Jeffrey RB Jr, Federle MP, Crass RA: Computed tomography of pancreatic trauma. *Radiology* 1983;147: 491–494.
15. Meyer DM, Thal ER, Weigelt JA, et al: The role of abdominal CT in the evaluation of stab wounds to the back. *J Trauma* 1989;29:1226–1230.
16. Phillips TF, Sclafani S, Goldstein A, et al: Use of contrast-enhanced CT enema in the management of penetrating trauma of the flank and back. *J Trauma* 1986;26:593–600.
17. Appleby JP, Nagy AG: Abdominal injuries associated with the use of seatbelts. *Am J Surg* 1989;157: 457–458.
18. Federle MP: Abdominal trauma: The role and impact of computed tomography. In Margulis A (ed): *Progress in Clinical Radiology*. Philadelphia: JB Lippincott, 1981.
19. Maull KI, Rozycki GS, Vinsant GO, et al: Retroperitoneal injuries: Pitfalls in diagnosis and management. *South Med J* 1987;80:1111–1115.

5

Technique for Surgical Exploration of the Abdomen

SCOTT B. FRAME, M.D., F.A.C.S.

Injuries to the structures contained in the retroperitoneum continue to constitute a major source of mortality in victims of both blunt and penetrating trauma (Table 5–1). This mortality rate has varied little over the course of the last 20 years. The manifestation of these injuries at the time of surgical exploration is a retroperitoneal hematoma. These hematomas arise from an organ or blood vessel lying posterior to the peritoneum lining the abdominal cavity. Obviously, the degree to which morbidity and mortality are affected by the presence of a retroperitoneal hematoma is determined by the source and quantity of the blood lost.

Not all retroperitoneal hematomas carry the same risk of injury to vital structures. Depending on the anatomic location, predictions may be made as to the possibility of which, if any, vital structures may be injured. The decision tree confronted intraoperatively will involve which retroperitoneal hematomas should be explored and which may be safely left intact. Some retroperitoneal hematomas are better left intact, because exploration raises the mortality rate (i.e., those associated with pelvic fractures).

The manner in which trauma patients are approached in the operating room will often determine their ultimate clinical course. It is imperative that the surgeon dealing with a patient undergoing exploration for abdominal trauma has a systematic approach to the operation so that injuries will not be missed. The missed injury at exploration is the nemesis of the surgeon and the creator of major morbidity and mortality for patients.[7,8] This is never truer than in the instance of missed retroperitoneal injuries. The retroperitoneum contains some of the most vital structures in the abdominal cavity, and occult injuries are the rule rather than the exception. Therefore, the surgeon must have an organized approach to the abdominal exploration so that a thorough evaluation of the retroperitoneum is made at every operation for abdominal trauma.

GENERAL CONSIDERATIONS

The approach to the trauma victim in the operating room should not differ significantly from one patient to the next. The same methodical approach should be carried out with each

Table 5–1   Mortality from Retroperitoneal Hematoma

REFERENCE	PERCENTAGE	NO. PATIENTS
Baylis et al[1]	18	50
Nick et al[2]	31	65
Allen et al[3]	24	75
Selivanov et al[4]	20	81
Henao and Aldrete[5]	19	203
Costa and Robbs[6]	13	106

patient so that the chances of surgical misadventure are minimized. If the surgeon develops a standard routine for the perioperative care of trauma victims, then he will lessen the opportunity that subtle findings may elude him.

It is very important that the surgeon and anesthesiologist cooperate in the care of the patient in the operating room. The patient must be quickly prepared for exploration once that decision has been reached. There is little to gain from extensive preoperative workup or consultation. It must be kept in mind that the definitive care of the trauma victim is surgical intervention. Delaying that definitive care with unnecessary laboratory tests, attempts at "stabilization," and concerns with preexisting medical conditions, will only serve to increase the chances for a bad outcome. While these delays are occurring, the patient is continuing to lose blood and may precipitously decompensate when no one is prepared to cope with it.

The patient should be placed in the supine position on the operating table. A broad-spectrum parenteral antibiotic is given preoperatively for prophylaxis in the event that hollow viscus injuries are present. Surgical skin preparation should be carried out while the surgeons are scrubbing. The author prefers a povidone-iodine scrub and spray, which should extend from the neck to the midthigh in every patient undergoing exploration for abdominal trauma. It is extremely important that the field should be widely prepped, as one must be prepared to cope with any eventuality. The chest must be ready to be entered, depending on intraoperative needs, and the vessels in the anterior thigh must be ready for surgical access (i.e., vascular control of the femoral artery, or harvesting of the saphenous vein for grafting). Any surgical preparation that is not this extensive is inadequate for a trauma exploration.

Prepping and draping are carried out prior to induction of anesthesia. Again, it is very important for the members of the team to cooperate fully in the care of the patient. Many trauma patients may appear stable, but will rapidly deteriorate on anesthetic induction. This deterioration may be extremely quick and catastrophic. If the surgeon is not prepared to begin exploration immediately and gain control of blood loss, the patient will be lost. The authors literally have knife in hand over a fully prepped and draped patient when the anesthesiologist induces the patient.

Prior to the commencement of celiotomy, it is also important to have available for immediate use a means for autologous, intraoperative blood transfusion. In this day and age of rising risks of blood transfusions, and the public's awareness of these risks, it is important to have the means for recycling the patient's shed blood during the course of the exploration. These devices take expertise to run and time to set up. Therefore it is imperative that this has been thought of in advance and appropriate preparations made. It has been recently shown[9] that shed blood may be safely infused back into the patient even in the presence of hollow viscus injuries with intra-abdominal contamination, so the use of these devices should not be avoided for any reason.

There should be no controversy on the proper incision to use when exploring the abdomen of the trauma patient. There is no way at this time to diagnose accurately every injury that may be present in any given patient. The surgeon must therefore be prepared to deal with any and all injuries that could possibly be found. In order to explore the trauma victim properly, every organ in the abdomen and retroperitoneum must be accessible. The only incision that offers this flexibility is a generous midline incision, extending from the xiphoid to the pubis, if necessary (Fig. 5–1). Assuming that injuries exist only in one portion of the abdomen and making an incision that limits the exploration to that portion of the celomic cavity will lead to missed injuries from incomplete exploration and the inability to deal properly with injuries present in other parts of the abdomen. It is the author's feeling that there is no place in trauma surgery for transverse, oblique, or any incisions other than the midline. Only this incision offers wide exposure for any and all structures, and by extending into the chest via a median sternotomy or thoracoabdominal incision, enables access to intrathoracic structures as well.

The philosophy that the surgeon must be prepared to handle any possible injury should be kept in mind when selecting equipment for the operative field. Remember that not only solid and hollow viscus injuries may be present, but vascular injuries may be present as well. Therefore, appropriate instruments should be readily available. It is wise to have the field equipped with two suction units, because large amounts of blood may have to be rapidly evacuated. Large numbers of laparotomy (lap) packs should also be available. The author likes to start an exploration with at least 50 lap packs already on the field.

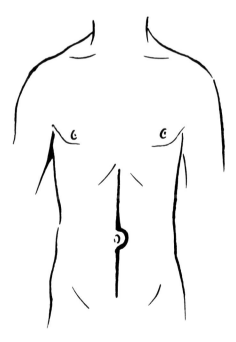

Figure 5–1.   Midline incision for trauma.

On entering the abdomen, large amounts of blood may be encountered. It is impossible to determine the source of the blood loss immediately. A helpful technique is to pack approximately ten lap packs into each quadrant of the abdomen. This serves a triple purpose. First, direct pressure is applied to all parts of the abdomen and this will aid in decreasing ongoing blood loss. Second, the evacuation of blood and clot is augmented and the abdomen becomes easier to explore. Lastly, each quadrant may be explored separately by removing the packs from each area, in turn, thereby aiding in establishing the source of hemorrhage.

If at any time during the exploration the patient should become hypotensive secondary to continued blood loss, the aorta should be occluded at the diaphragmatic hiatus. This maneuver will decrease ongoing blood loss and allow anesthesia to "catch up" with fluid resuscitation. Patients are often lost when the surgeon persists in pursuing an injury with rapid blood loss in a hypotensive patient. It is vastly preferable to control blood loss via direct pressure and aortic occlusion, and marshal one's resources. The proper instruments and equipment may be assembled and a plan outlined for approaching the injury. The anesthesia personnel may use the time to administer blood products and fluids to restore intravascular volume. In this fashion the surgeon does not continue to lose ground in his operative efforts. Only when all personnel are organized and the patient is as optimally fluid resuscitated as possible should the exploration and repair of injuries be continued.

A systematic exploration of all parts of the abdomen must be carried out in each patient. The method of exploration varies somewhat, depending on whether the patient is a victim of blunt or penetrating abdominal trauma. In the blunt abdominal trauma patient, all intra-abdominal and retroperitoneal structures are at risk for injury. In the penetrating abdominal trauma patient, the organs at risk for injury are limited somewhat by the tract of the injuring agent.

The exploration for blunt abdominal trauma must include a careful examination of all organs of the abdomen and retroperitoneum. The most commonly injured organs, liver and spleen, are examined first. Then the remainder of the intra-abdominal organs are explored. The stomach is examined, the small bowel is "run" (twice to ensure that nothing is missed), and a careful visual inspection of the colon is made. Attention is then turned to the structures of the retroperitoneum. The patient's small bowel should be eviscerated. This may be easily accomplished by simply "scooping" the viscera out of the abdomen toward the operating surgeon. In this fashion the root of the mesentery may be visualized and examined for the presence of hematomas.

A Kocher maneuver (Fig. 5–2) should always be performed in every exploration for blunt trauma. This enables excellent visualization of the second and third portions of the duodenum, as well as the opportunity to palpate carefully the head of the pancreas. The lesser sac must also be routinely entered through the gastrocolic ligament to allow careful inspection of the body and tail of the pancreas. Missed injuries to the duodenum or pancreas may be catastrophic, so care must be taken in *every* patient to avoid the morbidity and mortality of surgical shortcuts.

In penetrating abdominal wounds the exploration should include careful examination of all organs along the missile tract. Mobilization of any organ necessary to accomplish this should be done without hesitation. There are some caveats to this dictum that will be outlined later in the discussion of the approach to retroperitoneal hematomas. Again, it is essential that the entire small bowel be carefully examined to identify any injuries that may be present. Due to the mobility of the small bowel, even portions that are thought to

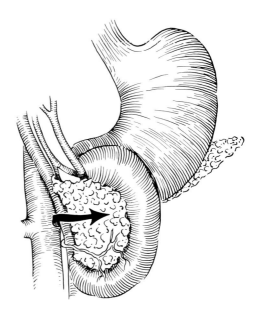

Figure 5–2. Kocher maneuver.

be distant from the missile tract may contain injuries. The redundancy and mobility of the transverse and sigmoid colons also mean that these organs warrant careful inspection in every exploration for penetrating trauma. Contusions on any hollow viscus should also be examined thoroughly, because they may herald occult perforations.

RETROPERITONEAL HEMATOMAS

Hematomas present in the retroperitoneum carry the potential of different problems based on their anatomic location. It is possible to divide the retroperitoneum arbitrarily into three portions (Fig. 5–3).[10] The first region (zone 1) is the upper central portion of the retroperitoneum. Anatomically, this extends from the diaphragmatic hiatus of the aorta and esophagus superiorly to the sacral promontory inferiorly, and lies between the kidneys, as the lateral boundaries. This region encompasses some of the most vital structures in the abdominal cavity. Included are the aorta, vena cava, renal vessels, portal vein, pancreas, and duodenum.

Zone 2 includes the right and left flanks, or the lateral retroperitoneum. This region includes the kidneys, the suprapelvic ureters, and the right and left mesocolons.

Zone 3 is the lower retroperitoneum and incorporates the pelvis. Structures included are the rectum, posterior bladder, and the pelvic ureters.

Retroperitoneal hematomas are usually diagnosed secondarily at exploration and may be associated with significant blood loss. Since they are rarely suspected prior to the time of exploration, it is important to have a plan prepared as to how these injuries will be dealt with if found. The management of retroperitoneal hematomas is often complex and is the source of controversy in the trauma literature.[11] The necessity of exploring retroperitoneal hematoma is determined by the method of injury (blunt versus penetrating), the anatomic location of the hematoma, and the expansion of the hematoma during the course of the operation.

Blunt abdominal trauma is not often the cause of major vascular injuries. Therefore the

67

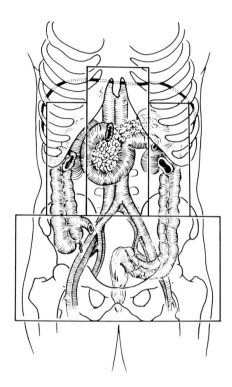

Figure 5–3. Retroperitoneal zones and their contents.

decision to explore retroperitoneal hematomas is usually based on the location and the expansile nature of the hematoma. Penetrating injuries, by contrast, do have a high incidence of major vascular trauma, and all zones 1 and 3 hematomas should be opened and explored.[12] Penetrating injuries in zone 2 are more controversial and may be selectively explored.

Due to the nature of the structures contained within the upper, central portion of the retroperitoneum, zone 1 injuries carry the highest morbidity and mortality. The high mortality is due to injuries to the aorta, vena cava, and celiac axis in the upper abdomen. Trauma to these structures just inferior to the diaphragm are difficult to expose and repair prior to exsanguination of the patient. Retroperitoneal hematomas in this area may also be present secondary to injuries of the posterior liver or the hepatic veins, both of which also carry high mortality. Greico and Perry[13] reported on two cases in which high, zone 1 hematomas resulted from transected thoracic aortas.

When a high, zone 1 hematoma is encountered at abdominal exploration, the surgeon has two choices as to how to proceed. Obviously, proximal vascular control of the aorta is the concern when approaching these injuries. It may be possible to gain control at the abdominal side of the aortic hiatus, but this is often very difficult to achieve and maintain. A superior method may be to proceed to an immediate left anterolateral thoracotomy and cross-clamp the thoracic aorta just superior to the diaphragm prior to entering the zone 1 hematoma. This will ensure adequate proximal control of the aorta and keeps the clamp out of the surgical field of repair.

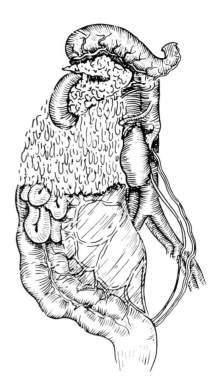

Figure 5–4. Mattox maneuver for exposure of the abdominal aorta.

Surgical exposure of the aorta has been facilitated by the introduction of the Mattox maneuver (Fig. 5–4).[14] This technique entails mobilization of the left and sigmoid colon, spleen, and left kidney enbloc and rotating the viscera on their vascular pedicles medially to expose the entire abdominal aorta. Since the introduction of this technique in 1974, it has become the standard method for exposing the aorta in most major trauma centers, including Houston[15] and Denver.[16] A more detailed discussion of the repair of these vascular injuries will be found in Chapter 11.

Access to the vena cava is achieved through the Cattell maneuver (Fig. 5–5).[17] This is a combined Kocher maneuver and mobilization of the right colon with medial rotation of the viscera. This offers excellent exposure of the entire vena cava. Proximal control of the vena cava is often difficult, if not impossible, to gain in injuries near the liver. Hematomas that extend up to the liver and into the portal triad should be approached with the aid of placement of a vena caval shunt (Fig. 5–6) prior to entering the hematoma. This is accomplished by extending the midline incision up into a median sternotomy to gain access to the right atrial appendage, through which the shunt is placed. Again, more details on the management of injuries to the vena cava will be found in Chapter 11.

Zone 1 hematomas are also associated with injuries to the pancreas and duodenum. Once major vascular injuries have been excluded, it is imperative that these structures be thoroughly examined for the presence of any injuries. Portal vein injuries will also produce hematomas in zone 1. They are frequently associated with injuries to the pancreas. As stated previously, a generous Kocher maneuver is imperative to explore the hematoma adequately

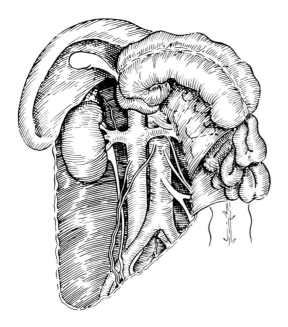

Figure 5–5.   Cattell maneuver for the exposure of the vena cava and the duodenum.

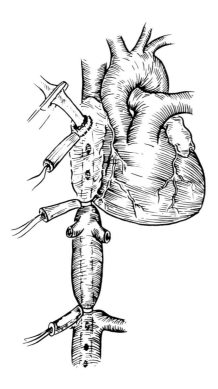

Figure 5–6.   Vena cava–right atrial shunt.

and the lesser sac must be entered to assess the pancreas. It cannot be overemphasized that these aspects of the exploration must not be neglected. Specifics on the management of injuries to the duodenum and pancreas are in Chapters 7 and 8, respectively.

Hematomas located in the lateral aspects of the upper retroperitoneum are classified as zone 2. These hematomas incorporate injuries to the kidneys. Management of these injuries has become controversial in the past several years. The routine exploration of these hematomas led to high rates of renal loss and mortality. More recent data have shown that some kidneys may be salvaged by not exploring the injuries. Approximately 95% of blunt renal injuries may be managed nonoperatively.[18] Penetrating renal trauma may be managed selectively. By carefully staging the injury and exploring only with specific indications,[19] approximately 50% of stab wounds and 15% of gunshot wounds may be managed nonoperatively.[20]

The intraoperative decision tree requires that an intravenous pyelogram has been performed. If this has not been done, then one should be performed on the operating table prior to the consideration of entering the hematoma. The information to be gained from pyelography is: (1) presence or absence of bilateral renal function; and (2) extravasation of contrast material from a renal unit. This information is combined with the operative findings to determine if exploration of the hematoma is warranted. Criteria that should lead to exploration are: (1) expanding or pulsatile hematoma; (2) evidence of extravasation on pyelography; or (3) pyelogram demonstrating loss of function on the side of the hematoma. It is important that vascular control of the kidney be obtained proximately prior to opening the hematoma. Opening the hematoma before vascular control has been gained has led to loss of the kidney in up to 75% of cases.[21] This proximal control may be obtained through the root of the mesentery, thereby leaving the hematoma intact. See Chapter 12 for further details on the treatment of injuries to the genitourinary system.

Zone 3 hematomas resulting from penetrating trauma should be explored without exception. Vascular injuries may be present and injuries to the rectum are common. Preoperative evaluation should have determined the presence of rectal injuries (see Chapter 3). Distal vascular control of distal iliac artery injuries may be obtained in the groin at the femoral artery (see Chapter 11). Rectal injuries are treated with proximal diversion, distal washout of the rectal stump, and presacral drainage. All three are required to minimize the chances of complications.[22,23] Direct suture closure of the rectal defect is not necessary as long as the three measures just mentioned are performed (see Chapter 10).

Pelvic fractures are by far the most common cause of zone 3 hematomas in blunt trauma. The management of these hematomas is extensively discussed in Chapter 13. Suffice it for now to make the general statement that these hematomas should never be entered at the time of initial exploration. These injuries carry a high mortality, which is made even worse by releasing the tamponade at surgery.

FEEDING JEJUNOSTOMY

It is the responsibility of the surgeon operating on the trauma patient to attempt to foresee potential problems in the postoperative period. Measures should be taken at the operating table to anticipate problems and institute early treatment to avoid them. Data are being rapidly gathered that indicate the beneficial effects of early postoperative enteral alimentation. Postoperative septic complications appear to be lessened by the early use of the gut. Enteral alimentation also is safer and less expensive than parenteral alimentation.

The authors strongly endorse the placement of a needle catheter jejunostomy (NCJ) at the time of the original exploration. The complications of the placement of NCJ through a Witzel tunnel are minimal, and it can be left in place through the patient's entire hospitalization. In this fashion it is ready to resume enteral alimentation if the clinical situation warrants. The authors usually pull the catheter out in the clinic after the patient has been discharged from the hospital and is doing well at home.

Moore et al[24] have attempted to define those patients in whom placement of a NCJ should be performed. They have defined an Abdominal Trauma Index (ATI) and advocate the placement of NCJ if the ATI is above 15. If the ATI is above 25, immediate enteral alimentation is begun, and if the score is above 40, parenteral alimentation is immediately begun and transition to enteral done at the earliest possible time. The NCJ can be used to provide enteral alimentation even in the presence of an ileus. Intolerance of the feedings is uncommon and usually occurs when the serum albumin is below 2.8 mg/dl. Exogenous albumin can be given to correct the albumin deficit and eliminate the intolerance problem. The authors strongly endorse these guidelines and are currently following them for all our trauma patients.

SUMMARY

The successful surgical management of the patient with retroperitoneal injuries demands that an organized approach be taken for the exploration. Retroperitoneal hematomas are the manifestation of injuries to structures contained within the retroperitoneum. Initial exploration of the abdomen should be directed not only at injuries to intra-abdominal organs, but also to identifying these hematomas. After retroperitoneal hematomas have been found, their management is determined by mechanism of injury, location, and intraoperative expansion.

All retroperitoneal hematomas resulting from penetrating trauma should be opened and thoroughly explored. The only exceptions to this rule are those hematomas in zone 2 that do not meet the previously stated criteria for exploration.

Retroperitoneal hematomas secondary to blunt trauma have a more complex decision tree to follow. All zone 1 hematomas should be opened and explored because they carry a 65% incidence of vascular injuries.[25] Also, damage to the duodenum and pancreas must be ruled out. Zone 2 injuries are explored utilizing the same criteria as outlined previously in this chapter. Zone 3 injuries are left alone if at all possible at the initial exploration. These hematomas are approached surgically only when all other available measures have failed to control ongoing hemorrhage.

A NCJ should be placed in all patients except those with minor injuries. Early enteral alimentation should be pursued in all patients in which the clinical situation allows it.

REFERENCES

1. Baylis SM, Lansing EH, Glas WW: Traumatic retroperitoneal hematoma. *Am J Surg* 1962;103:477–480.
2. Nick WV, Zollinger RW, Pace WG: Retroperitoneal hemorrhage after blunt abdominal trauma. *J Trauma* 1967;7:652–659.

3. Allen RE, Eastman BA, Halter BL, Conolly WB: Retroperitoneal hemorrhage secondary to blunt trauma. *Am J Surg* 1969;118:558–561.
4. Selivanov V, Chi HS, Alverdy JC, Morris JA, Shelton GF: Mortality in retroperitoneal hematoma. *J Trauma* 1984;24:1022–1027.
5. Henao F, Aldrete JS: Retroperitoneal hematomas of traumatic origin. *Surg Gynecol Obstet* 1985;161: 106–116.
6. Costa M, Robbs JV: Management of retroperitoneal haematoma following penetrating trauma. *Br J Surg* 1985;72:662–664.
7. Scalea TM, Phillips TF, Goldstein AS, Sclafani JA, Duncan AO, Atweh NA, Shaftan GW: Injuries missed at operation: Nemesis of the trauma surgeon. *J Trauma* 1988;28:962–967.
8. Enderson BL, Maull KI: Missed injuries: The trauma surgeon's nemesis. *Surg Clin North Am* 1991;71: 399–417.
9. Timberlake GA, McSwain NE: Autotransfusion of blood contaminated by enteric contents: A potentially life-saving measure in the massively hemorrhaging trauma patient? *J Trauma* 1988;28:855–857.
10. Kudsk KA, Sheldon GF: Retroperitoneal hematoma. In Blaisdell FW, Trunkey DD (eds): *Abdominal Trauma*. New York: Thieme-Stratton, 1982, pp 279–293.
11. Gill W, Champion HR, Long WB, Austin EA, Cowley RA: Controversial aspects of abdominal trauma. *J R Coll Surg* 1975;20:174–197.
12. Steichen FM, Dargan EL, Pearlman DM, Weil PH: The management of retroperitoneal hematoma secondary to penetrating injuries. *Surg Gynecol Obstet* 1966;123:581–591.
13. Greico JG, Perry JF: Retroperitoneal hematoma following trauma: Its clinical significance. *J Trauma* 1980;20:733–736.
14. Mattox KL, McCollum WB, Beall AC, Jordan GL, Debakey ME: Management of penetrating injuries of the suprarenal aorta. *J Trauma* 1975;15:808–815.
15. Accola KD, Feliciano DV, Mattox KL, Bitondo CG, Burch JM, Beall AC, Jordan GL: Management of injuries to the suprarenal aorta. *Am J Surg* 1987;154:613–618.
16. Millikan JS, Moore EE: Critical factors in determining mortality from abdominal aortic trauma. *Surg Gynecol Obstet* 1985;160:313–316.
17. Cattell RB, Braasch JW: A technique for the exposure of the third and fourth portions of the duodenum. *Surg Gynecol Obstet* 1960;111:379–380.
18. Peterson NE: Intermediate-degree blunt renal trauma. *J Trauma* 1977;17:425–435.
19. Carroll PR, McAninch JW: Operative indications in penetrating renal trauma. *J Trauma* 1985;25:587–593.
20. McAninch JW: Genitourinary trauma. In Mattox KL, Moore EE, Feliciano DV (eds): *Trauma*. Norwalk, CT: Appleton and Lange, 1988, pp 537–552.
21. McAninch JW, Carroll PR: Renal trauma: Preservation through improved vascular control—a refined approach. *J Trauma* 1982;22:285–290.
22. Burch JM, Feliciano DV, Mattox K: Colostomy and drainage for civilian rectal injuries: Is that all? *Ann Surg* 1989;209:600–611.
23. Shannon FL, Moore EE, Moore FA, McCroskey BL: Value of distal colon washout in civilian rectal trauma—reducing gut bacterial translocation. *J Trauma* 1988;28:989–994.
24. Moore EE, Dunn EL, Moore JB, et al: Penetrating abdominal trauma index. *J Trauma* 1981;21:439–445.
25. Attard J: Upper retroperitoneal injuries. *Br J Surg* 1971;58:55–60.

6

Esophagus

NORMAN E. McSWAIN, JR., M.D., F.A.C.S.

Although the esophagus is predominantly a thoracic structure, its lower segment lies in a difficult portion of the abdomen in which to gain access. In addition, it is totally retroperitoneal throughout its short course in the abdomen. The lower 2 cm are retroperitoneal, and as with the other retroperitoneal gastrointestinal GI tract structures, it is not protected with peritoneum, which will either produce peritonitis to improve diagnosis or enhance healing after an injury. Therefore steps must be taken to diagnose accurately the injury in its acute phase. The usual preoperative diagnostic techniques used for the trauma patient are not helpful for these injuries. Repair means dealing with mainly a muscular organ, one that does not hold sutures particularly well, and one that must be adequately protected postoperatively to prevent leakage.

ANATOMY

Although the esophagus begins as the hypopharynx, then divides into the trachea and the esophagus in the upper neck, its course as the abdominal retroperitoneal structure begins as it passes through the crux of the diaphragm and ends with its attachment to the stomach. This portion of the esophagus is from 2 to 7 cm in length and is covered only on its anterior surface with peritoneum, or not covered at all. The sides and posterior surface are not protected by serosa, although occasionally the peritoneum may extend down laterally to provide partial coverage (Fig. 6–1). As it joins the stomach, its actual point of entry is not at the top but on the medial border. This unique anatomic location allows the stomach to be used to protect injuries of the lower esophagus (Fig. 6–2).

The blood supply to this portion comes from below through the left gastric artery. The venous drainage goes in the same direction (Fig. 6–3).

As the esophagus descends from the thoracic cavity to the abdominal cavity, it crosses through the diaphragm's fibromuscular attachments to the vertebral bodies known as crura. In penetrating trauma these structures may be damaged and require repair; therefore they must be closely inspected. The esophagus lies in close approximation to the aorta and near the vena cava. Access is easy both through the thorax and the abdomen; however, because of the possibility of associated injuries in the abdomen, the abdominal approach is desirable.

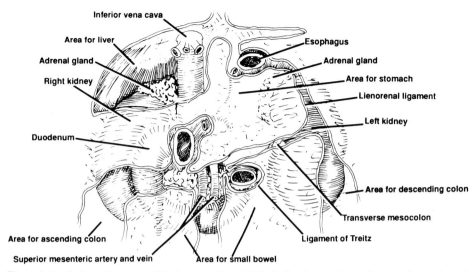

Figure 6–1. Peritoneal coverage of the lower esophageal is limited to the anterior esophagus at the esophageal gastric junction.

ASSESSMENT

Assessment of the esophagus preoperatively is difficult. Endoscopy, of course, can provide visualization; however, flexible endoscopy is not as accurate for finding small defects as rigid endoscopy. Both a rigid esophagoscope and radiographic survey are necessary to rule out such injuries completely. Rigid esophagoscopy on a trauma patient may not be practical, since it does require time and is a technique that would require general anesthesia in this setting. Following the general rule that trauma that penetrates deeply enough to cause

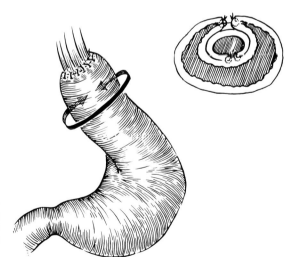

Figure 6–2. The upper portion of the fundus is actually above the esophageal entrance at the lesser curvature. A wrap of the fundus around the esophagus to protect a repair is anatomically simple.

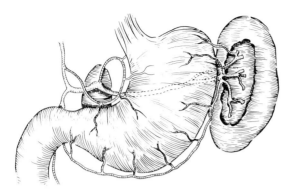

Figure 6–3. Blood supply of the esophagus is via the left gastric artery.

possible injury to the esophagus should be explored because of the possibility of associated injuries, such diagnostic maneuvers are only required if open exploration does not completely rule out an injury.

Blunt trauma to the esophagus is rare. Beal et al[1] reported in 1988 only 96 cases of blunt trauma in the literature (including five of their own) since 1900. Of those cases, 82% were in the cervical and upper thoracic portions. Lack of symptoms contributed to a high mortality and morbidity rate. Glatterer et al[2] reported on 26 patients with both blunt and penetrating trauma to the esophagus. Only one of these injuries was to the abdominal esophagus (4%). Symbas et al[3] reported in 1980 on 48 injuries over a 15-year period from Grady Hospital. Seven, or 15%, were in the abdomen, the rest in the cervical or thoracic part of the organ. Trauma to the thoracic and cervical esophagus represents special conditions; these are not part of the retroperitoneum and therefore are not discussed in this work.

Even though the injury is rare, the clinician must always be suspicious. Atter et al[4] found that the mortality rate increased from 16% to 52% if the patients were not diagnosed in the first 24 hours.

MANAGEMENT

Once injury to the esophagus has been identified, all areas of possible injury must be exposed. This can be accomplished either through a thoracic incision, with an associated incision in the diaphragm, or by pulling the injured portion into the abdominal cavity from the abdominal incision. Pulling the esophagus into the abdominal cavity mandates two prerequisites: (1) the esophagus is not totally transected and traction on the stomach will not produce a total transection; and (2) the esophagus has been mobilized high enough into the mediastinum so that it can be pulled into the abdomen with adequate length for repair.

The peritoneum is incised over the esophagus, blunt finger dissection is used to mobilize the esophagus in the mediastinum (Fig. 6–4). After mobilization a Penrose drain can be passed around the gastroesophageal junction to apply traction during closure (Fig. 6–5). The injury should be repaired in two layers with interrupted nonabsorbable sutures, if possible. The stomach is wrapped around the esophagus to cover and protect the repair. The suture technique is similar to the fundoplication operation (Nissen repair) done for esophageal reflux.

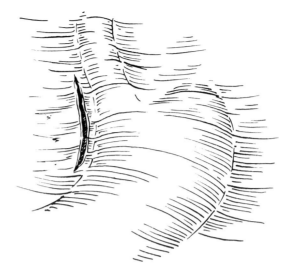

Figure 6–4. Incision of the peritoneum overlying the gastroesophageal junction allows access to the esophagus.

It is not necessary to divert the secretions from the salivary glands by cervical esophagotomy but it is helpful to pass a nasogastric tube into the lower esophagus just above the injury to remove secretions and to prevent pressure buildup at the site of the repair. A gastrostomy tube is used to decompress the stomach. This prevents both a pressure buildup below the injury and reflux. A feeding jejunostomy should also be placed to provide postoperative nutrition (Fig. 6–6).

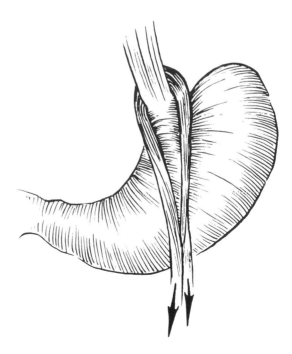

Figure 6–5. Penrose drain is passed around the esophagus to provide better traction and visibility of the upper esophagus.

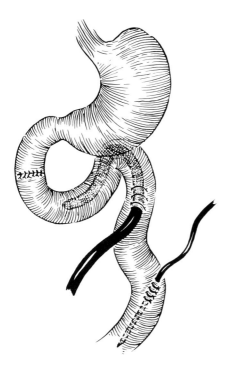

Figure 6–6.   Feeding jejunostomy provides nutrition while the esophageal repair heals. Placement of the tube is the same as previously described for duodenal injuries.

SUMMARY

Injury to the retroperitoneal esophagus is extremely rare. The majority of injuries are penetrating etiology. Injuries may be difficult to diagnose, and exposure for repair is not easily obtained. However, delayed diagnosis increases morbidity and mortality. Surgical repair is best protected with adequate postoperative decompression and the stomach is wrapped around the suture line.

REFERENCES

1.   Beal SL, Pottmeyer DW, Spisso JM: Esophageal perforation following external blunt trauma. *J Trauma* 1988;28:1425–1432.
2.   Glatterer MS Jr, Toon RS, Ellestad C, McFee AS, Rogers W, Mack JW, Trinkle JK, Grover FL: Management of blunt and penetrating external esophageal trauma. *J Trauma* 1985;25:784–792.
3.   Symbas PN, Hatcher CR Jr, Vlasis SE: Esophageal gunshot injuries. *Ann Surg* 1980;191:703–707.
4.   Atter S, Hankins JR, Suter CM, Coughlin TR, Sequeira A, McLaughlin JS: Esophageal perforation: A therapeutic challenge. *Ann Thorac Surg* 1990;50:45–49.

7

Duodenal Trauma

SCOTT B. FRAME, M.D., F.A.C.S.

The duodenum lies deep within the abdomen in the upper, central portion of the retroperitoneum. It is protected on the posterior aspect by the vertebral column and the thick paraspinous muscles. Anteriorly, the second, third, and fourth portions lie deep to the remainder of the upper, intraabdominal organs. Due to this relatively well-protected position, injuries to the duodenum are not common, occurring in approximately 5% of patients with intra-abdominal injuries.[1] The first report of a successful treatment of a duodenal injury was by Herzel in 1896.[2] He described the primary suture repair of a patient with a duodenal wound who survived the injury.

Penetrating trauma accounts for the majority of duodenal injuries, with 86%, and only 14% of injuries being due to blunt trauma.[3–8] The incidence of penetrating duodenal injuries has been on the rise over the last 20 years. This rise is probably attributable to the increased use of guns in our violent society. When knives were the most common wounding agent, the deep structures of the abdomen and retroperitoneum were out of reach and only rarely injured.

Duodenal injuries are commonly associated with other intra-abdominal trauma. Ninety to 95% of duodenal wounds have associated injuries.[9] The most commonly associated organ is the liver, followed closely by major vascular structures, colon, pancreas, and stomach. Extrahepatic biliary injuries are also common due to the close anatomic relationship of the two structures. Due to the high degree of force required to injure the duodenum in blunt trauma, patients most often have extra-abdominal injuries as well.

Mortality from duodenal wounds is directly related to the presence of the associated injuries and ranges from 13 to 28%.[4–8] The most common cause of early mortality is uncontrolled hemorrhage. Late deaths are attributable to the associated injuries and sepsis, with sepsis implicated in at least one quarter of the deaths. Blunt trauma to the duodenum has a higher mortality than penetrating, 16.7 to 7.5%.[4] This difference is most likely secondary to both delay in diagnosis and higher incidence of associated injuries commonly found in blunt trauma.

Morbidity from duodenal injuries is primarily related to the incidence of fistula formation after repair. This rate ranges from 2 to 14%.[4–8] The remainder of complications are related to the associated injuries.

DIAGNOSIS

The diagnosis of penetrating injuries to the duodenum usually comes as an intraoperative finding. During the exploration of the abdomen for a penetrating wound, particularly of the right upper quadrant, careful examination of the duodenum must be carried out. The author believes that all stab wounds of the abdomen that are proven through local exploration to penetrate the anterior rectus sheath should undergo celiotomy. The diagnostic accuracy of peritoneal lavage has not been proven through well-controlled, prospective trials, and the study has been demonstrated to be insensitive to retroperitoneal injuries. The author also believes that routine exploration of all gunshot wounds of the abdomen is the standard of care for this mechanism of injury.

The diagnosis of blunt injuries to the duodenum is more difficult, especially if the injury is isolated. The most common scenario is that duodenal injury is found at exploration when associated injuries have precipitated celiotomy. If there is an obvious abdominal wound, peritoneal signs on examination, or evidence of intra-abdominal hemorrhage, the patient should be taken for immediate exploratory celiotomy.

For blunt abdominal trauma, diagnostic peritoneal lavage remains the diagnostic test of choice. A positive lavage will indicate the need for urgent exploratory celiotomy. However, as previously stated in Chapter 3, a negative lavage does not exclude the presence of retroperitoneal trauma. This is particularly true of duodenal and pancreatic injuries. A high index of suspicion is essential when the mechanism of injury makes the chance of duodenal injury likely.

Laboratory tests are of little value in the diagnosis of duodenal trauma. The determination of the serum amylase has been touted as a helpful test, but has not proven to be accurate enough to base a diagnosis on. The serum amylase is elevated in only 50% of patients with duodenal injury.[6,8] The use of amylase isoenzymes has also not been of diagnostic benefit.[10,11] The measurement of the amylase from the effluent of the peritoneal lavage is likewise not helpful as an immediate determination. However, the finding of a rising amylase on repeat lavage is a strong indication of either pancreatic or duodenal injury.

The upright chest and abdominal radiographs may give valuable information, as outlined in Chapter 3. Evidence of retroperitoneal air (Fig. 7–1) is strong evidence for the presence of a duodenal disruption. Free air under the diaphragm indicates a hollow viscus perforation, from either a peritoneal organ or intra-abdominal perforation of a retroperitoneal organ. Air in the biliary tree of the post-trauma patient is also an indication of retroperitoneal injury, particularly of the duodenum. Other, nonspecific signs of retroperitoneal trauma include scoliosis to the right, obliteration of the psoas shadow, and retroperitoneal air around the kidney. These findings have been reported in more than 90% of patients with duodenal trauma.[12] Air may also be injected through the nasogastric tube prior to obtaining a flat plate of the abdomen. This may more clearly demonstrate retroperitoneal air in a patient suspected of having a duodenal wound.

An upper gastrointestinal contrast study may help to diagnose a duodenal injury in the patient in whom there is a high level of suspicion. A water-soluble contrast medium should be utilized in these patients to avoid the dense inflammatory reaction produced by the extravasation of barium. The patient should be placed in the right lateral decubitus position for the performance of this test to maximize the duodenal concentration of the contrast and improve the accuracy of the examination. A negative water-soluble contrast

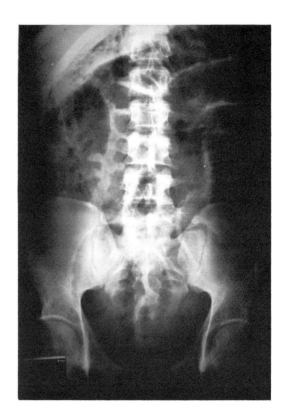

Figure 7–1. Abdominal radiograph demonstrating retroperitoneal air secondary to duodenal rupture from blunt trauma.

study should be followed by a barium study to exclude conclusively a duodenal perforation. Small leaks may be missed by the water-soluble contrast, but picked up on the barium study.

In centers where the reliability of the test has been confirmed and the expertise exists for the proper interpretation of the study, the computed tomograph is probably the best diagnostic aid for retroperitoneal trauma. The study must be performed with both oral and intravenous contrast. The use of computed tomography in retroperitoneal trauma is the topic of Chapter 4.

OPERATIVE MANAGEMENT

As explained in Chapter 5, all zone 1 retroperitoneal hematomas should be carefully explored when found during celiotomy. The duodenum must be mobilized via the Kocher maneuver to examine it adequately for damage. Other signs found at operation that mandate careful exploration of the duodenum include: crepitus or bile staining along the lateral margin of the duodenum; retroperitoneal edema, petechiae or fat necrosis in the retroperitoneum or right mesocolon; or retroperitoneal phlegmon.[13] It may be necessary to mobilize the right colon in the Cattell maneuver to visualize the third and fourth portions of the duodenum adequately.[14]

Simple Lacerations

The majority of injuries to the duodenum are simple lacerations that can be repaired primarily. Approximately 70 to 85% of duodenal injuries are amenable to simple duodenorrhaphy (Fig. 7–2).[8,15] It is important, especially in penetrating trauma, to examine the posterior wall of the duodenum to look for exit wounds. Again, most of these wounds can be closed with simple suture repair. Care must be taken not to compromise the lumen of the duodenum when performing the repair. This is critically important in the pyloric channel region.

   Closure may be accomplished with either a one- or two-layer closure. The important point is to observe meticulous technique. Knife wounds normally make clean lacerations, with minimal nonviable tissue present along the edges. This is not the case with blunt tears or gunshot wounds. There may be extensive nonviable tissue present along the wound edges. It is critically important to perform adequate debridement. The wound that is closed without proper debridement is doomed to break down and leak. It must be remembered that the closure of a hollow viscus wound is no different from any bowel anastomosis, and the same principles apply. The suture line must be made without tension and there must be good blood supply to the anastomosis. If nonviable tissue is not debrided, the suture line will not have an adequate blood supply and failure is predetermined. Debridement may require resection and this should be performed rather than placing sutures through nonviable tissue.

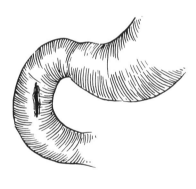

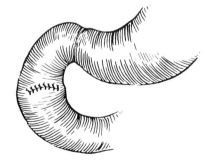

Figure 7–2.   Simple duodenorrhaphy.

Complex Duodenal Injuries with Loss of Wall

Some of the most severe injuries to the duodenum involve the loss of a portion of the duodenal wall. These injuries present extremely difficult problems to solve for the trauma surgeon and require special techniques for repair. When the injury involves only the lateral wall of the duodenum, primary repair may still be possible. It is important to mobilize the entire duodenum completely in these cases so that as much bowel as possible is available for closure. Some compromise of the lumen can be accepted, but it is important to ensure that the suture line is not made under too much tension. When closure cannot be made without compromising the lumen too much or placing too much tension on the suture line, then special techniques must be performed to gain closure of the defect.

Side-to-side or end-to-side duodenojejunostomy may be used to secure a sound closure of a large defect (Fig. 7–3).[16] The danger exists that jejunal contents may reflux into the duodenum, but this is rarely a problem. To avoid the possibility of reflux, the anastomosis can be made using a Roux-en-Y limb of jejunum brought up to the duodenum.

A vascularized pedicle of jejunum may also be used to close the wound (Fig. 7–4).[17] This procedure gives an excellent closure, but is more complicated and time consuming. It should be reserved for the stable patient with minimal associated injuries who can tolerate the additional operative time required. This technique involves the creation of the pedicled jejunal patch, suture of the patch over the duodenal wound, and a jejunojejunostomy to reestablish small bowel continuity. Care must be taken to avoid twisting the jejunal patch on its pedicle, so as not to compromise the vascular supply.

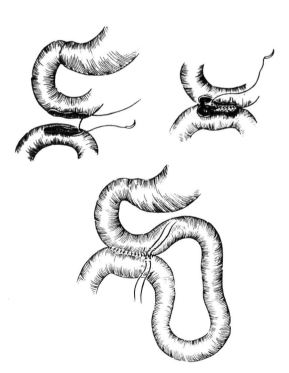

Figure 7–3. Duodenojejunostomy.

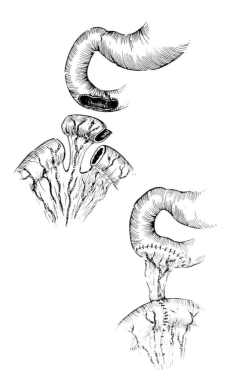

Figure 7–4.   Vascularized jejunal mucosal pedicle patch.

The defect may also be closed using a serosal patch formed from a loop of jejunum (Fig. 7–5).[18] This type of repair does not require the formation of a formal anastomosis. A loop of intact jejunum is sutured over the defect to seal the wound. This exposes the serosal surface of the jejunum to the contents of the duodenum and causes a dense serositis. This reaction may result in the formation of a fistula between the jejunum and the duodenum. This rarely causes problems because it creates the same situation as a properly performed duodenojejunostomy.

The combination of a primary repair with a covering serosal patch has not been shown to be any more effective than using primary repair alone.[19,20]

Segmental resection with primary end-to-end anastomosis of the duodenum may be necessary to achieve adequate debridement of devitalized tissue (Fig. 7–6). This can be accomplished in all portions of the duodenum except the second. The presence of the ampulla of Vater and the shared blood supply with the pancreas in this region make resection impossible. In these cases the more complex repairs, as already described, should be used. Rarely, pancreaticoduodenectomy may be necessary for injuries in the second portion involving damage to the ampulla, uncontrollable hemorrhage from the pancreaticoduodenal vascular arcade, or a devascularized duodenum.[21]

The use of tube decompression of the duodenum is the source of some controversy. Both Stone and Fabian,[7] and Hasson et al[22] advocate the routine use of tube decompression for duodenal repair. In the series by Stone and Fabian one fistula developed in 237 patients treated with duodenorrhaphy and tube decompression, whereas fistulas formed in eight of 44 patients treated without tube decompression. Similar results were cited by

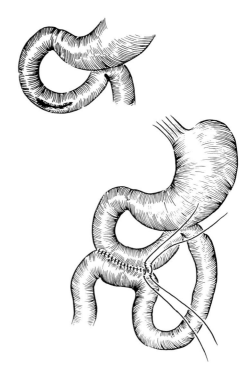

Figure 7–5. Jejunal serosal patch.

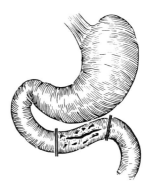

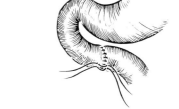

Figure 7–6. Segmental resection with primary end-to-end anastomosis.

Hasson et al in a review of several series of duodenal repairs. The fistula rate with tube decompression was 2.3% compared with a fistula rate of 11.8% without decompression. If the decompression tube was placed through the duodenal wall, the fistula rate was 19.4%. On the other side is the report of Snyder et al,[8] who found no difference in the morbidity rate in simple closure with or without tube decompression.

Tube decompression may be accomplished in several different fashions. A nasal tube may be placed at the time of surgery through the pylorus into the duodenum. A tube may be brought out through the lateral duodenal wall in proximity to the injury. However, as pointed out previously, Hasson et al found their highest fistula rate when the tube was brought out through the duodenal wall. The tube may also be placed retrograde into the duodenum through a more distally placed Witzel tunnel jejunostomy (Fig. 7–7). The latter method is probably the most preferred technique for achieving decompression when deemed necessary. The author does not routinely use decompression, but in severe injuries when it is required, the retrograde method is used.

Snyder et al[8] proposed criteria for establishing the severity of the injury to the duodenum. These criteria may be used to determine which patients have severe injuries and require more complex procedures, rather than simple closure. All patients with stab wounds to the second or third portions of the duodenum were placed into the mild injury group unless one or more of the other factors were present.

The results of this study demonstrated the increased morbidity and mortality rates of the injuries classified as severe by their criteria. Mild injuries had a mortality rate of zero and a fistula rate of 2%. In those injuries classified as severe, the rates were 6 and 10%, respectively. It is strongly recommended that when the defect is too large for primary

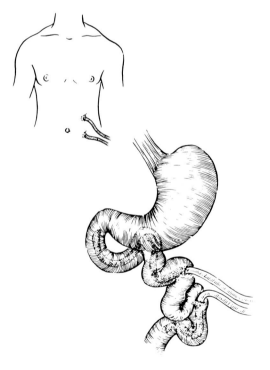

Figure 7–7. Retrograde duodenostomy tube.

closure or meets Snyder's criteria for a severe injury, a complex repair is appropriate. Serious consideration should be given to tube decompression when a complex repair is performed.

Transection of the Duodenum

If the duodenum is totally transected, the preferred method of treatment is debridement and primary anastomosis. As stated previously, this is possible in all portions of the duodenum except the second. Extensive tissue loss may result in a defect that cannot be closed without undue tension on the suture line. If this is the case and the defect is distal to the ampulla of Vater, then the distal end should be closed and an anastomosis made to the jejunum with the proximal end (Fig. 7–8). If the situation exists proximal to the ampulla, then the duodenal stump is closed and a Billroth II antrectomy with gastrojejunostomy is the procedure of choice. Complete transection in the second portion of the duodenum involving the ampulla usually requires that a pancreaticoduodenectomy be carried out.

Duodenal Diverticulization and Exclusion

The use of duodenal diverticulization was popularized by Berne et al[23] in 1974 (Fig. 7–9). The purpose of this procedure is to effect repair of the duodenum and then isolate the

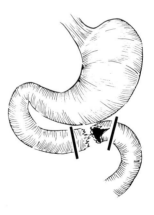

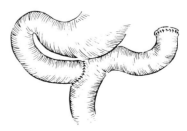

Figure 7–8. Duodenojejunostomy for distal duodenal transection.

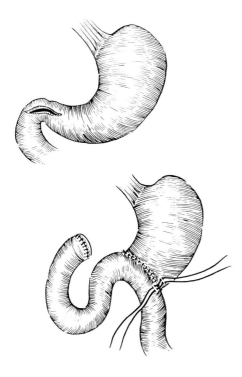

Figure 7–9. Duodenal diverticulization.

duodenum from the gastrointestinal flow. If a fistula does occur, it will be an end fistula and not a lateral one. Also, since the duodenum is isolated from enteric contents, it becomes a low-pressure area. Biliary and pancreatic secretions continue to flow through the area, but these can normally be managed and spontaneous closure of the fistula is almost assured.

The technique calls for the performance of a gastric antrectomy, formation of a gastrojejunostomy, closure of the duodenal stump, repair of the duodenal wound, and placement of a distal jejunal decompression catheter. Truncal vagotomy may be used with the procedure, and the author advocates its inclusion. Biliary drainage may also be added to the procedure if the clinical situation warrants it.

This technique has begun to lose proponents over the last several years as the technique of pyloric exclusion has gained favor. The purpose of the diverticulization procedure was to divert enteric flow to allow the duodenal repair to heal. This diversion does not have to be permanent to achieve the same purpose. In 1977, the group at Baylor in Houston described the pyloric exclusion procedure to create a temporary duodenal diversion, which is technically easier to perform than the diverticulization procedure (Fig. 7–10).[24] This operation consists of repair of the duodenal wound, formation of a gastrojejunostomy, and closure of the pylorus through the gastrostomy made for the creation of the gastrojejunostomy.

Originally, the closure of the pylorus was performed with a catgut suture. Jordan's group[1] in Houston now uses a Prolene® suture, and closure with staples has also been performed. The procedure was initially devised to be temporary with the catgut dissolving and the pylorus reopening with reinstitution of normal enteric flow. These authors have

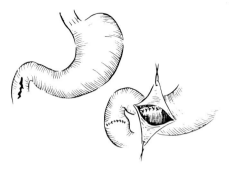

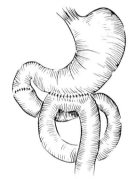

Figure 7–10. Pyloric exclusion for duodenal diversion.

found that the pylorus is extremely difficult to permanently occlude by any technique. They have studied over 50 patients and found that the pylorus is usually open within 3 weeks. Two closures with polypropylene sutures were documented to have remained closed for several weeks, one still closed at 37 days and the second at 53 days. One closure performed with staples was documented to have remained for several months.

Currently, those authors advocate the use of Prolene® sutures to close the pylorus. In some of the patients in whom catgut or even Dexon® was used, reopening of the pylorus occurred within 2 weeks, a period deemed too short for safe healing of the duodenum.

The addition of a vagotomy to the procedure is not advocated. The time spent performing a truncal vagotomy in these critically injured patients is not worth the theoretical benefit. When properly performed, the procedure is not ulcerogenic and should not result in a higher ulcer rate than that found in the normal population. An extremely important part of the operation is making absolutely certain that the pylorus is occluded at the proper position. No portion of the antrum must be included in the closure, since this results in retained antrum and the formation of an ulcerogenic preparation. If this tenet is observed, the rate of marginal ulceration has been shown to be 3% in 135 patients in whom the procedure has been performed.[1] This rate does not exceed the incidence of ulcer found in the normal population.

The treatment of complex injuries to the duodenum is controversial. As has been shown in the discussion thus far, there are several acceptable means to manage any given wound. In the Houston series of 135 patients using the duodenal exclusion procedure in severe duodenal wounds, the results have been excellent. There were only two deaths attributable to the duodenal wound (overall mortality rate, 22%) and the fistula formation rate was reduced from 6% in an earlier series to 2% in the more recent series using pyloric exclusion.[1,9,25]

The two described diversion techniques have an excellent record, as measured by their morbidity and mortality rates. It must be kept in mind that these techniques are not required in the majority of patients with duodenal injuries. As previously pointed out, up to 85% of wounds may be managed via simple closure with or without the addition of tube decompression. In the remaining patients more complex procedures need to be considered. In only 10 to 15% of patients will duodenal diversion be necessary.[26] These complex techniques should be reserved for those patients with the most severe duodenal injuries.

Pancreaticoduodenectomy

Recent reports by Oreskovich and Carrico,[21] McKone et al,[27] and Heimansohn et al[28] have demonstrated the safety of performing pancreaticoduodenectomy in carefully selected patients with duodenal or pancreatic trauma (Fig. 7–11). Both of these reports cited a zero mortality rate and an acceptable complication rate. In the 19 patients reported on in the combined series there was one pancreatic fistula and two patients with pancreatic insufficiency.

McKone et al proposed the following indications for the performance of the procedure: (1) extensive devitalization of the head of the pancreas and duodenum so that other measures of treatment are likely to fail because of loss of duodenal vascularity or the almost certain

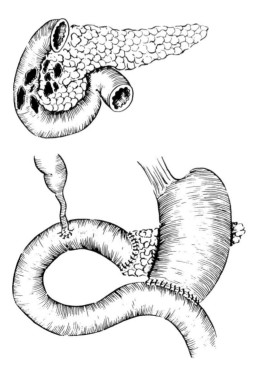

Figure 7–11.   Pancreaticoduodenectomy.

postoperative occurrence of a pancreatic fistula; (2) ductal disruption in the pancreatic head in association with injury to the duodenum or common bile duct; (3) injury to the ampulla of Vater, especially when there is disruption of the main pancreatic duct from the duodenum; (4) uncontrollable bleeding from the head of the pancreas; or (5) retropancreatic portal vein injury.

Drainage

Routine drainage of simple duodenal injuries treated with primary closure is not only unnecessary, but may be harmful by increasing the incidence of intra-abdominal sepsis by acting as a conduit for the introduction of bacteria into the peritoneal cavity. Routine drainage is to be vigorously discouraged. Severe duodenal injuries requiring the more complex procedures should have accompanying drainage. When drainage is performed, the method of choice is via closed suction drains, preferably of the silicone or Silastic variety. The author strongly condemns the use of Penrose drains for use within the abdomen, no matter what the indications. These passive drains act as a portal of entry for bacteria while offering nothing in active removal of fluid collections.

COMPLICATIONS

As with any multitrauma patient the list of possible complications is extensive. However, there are only two complications that are directly related to the repair of the duodenal injury. These are duodenal fistula formation and duodenal obstruction.

Duodenal Fistula

The most feared complication of duodenal repair is formation of a duodenal fistula. The older literature cited mortality rates of 50 to 75% for lateral duodenal fistulas. This high mortality rate stems from the lack of methods to prevent and treat intra-abdominal sepsis, and the lack of understanding of the metabolic consequences of the fistula. Currently, the reported incidence of duodenal fistula in a collected series of 1563 patients was 3 to 12%.[25] The late mortality directly related to the duodenal injury, exclusive of associated injuries, was less than 1%.

It is often said that the best defense is a good offense. This philosophy is never truer than when applied to medicine. The best treatment for a complication is to prevent the complication in the first place. In duodenal injuries this means carefully evaluating the injury and performing the most appropriate procedure for the wound present. As previously pointed out, adequate debridement is essential in order to ensure the best possible outcome. In severe injuries requiring complex reconstructive procedures, the use of closed suction drainage should be encouraged. This will aid in forming a controlled duodenal fistula if one develops. In this manner peritonitis is avoided and skin protection is easier to accomplish.

It is important in the immediate postoperative period to maintain fluid and electrolyte balance through vigorous intravenous fluid therapy. The majority of duodenal fistulas will close with nasogastric suction, proper drainage, and intravenous alimentation. If a feeding jejunostomy has been placed at surgery, it serves as an ideal route for the provision of enteral alimentation, thereby avoiding the complications of parenteral alimentation. If the patient has had duodenal diverticulization or exclusion performed, then the oral route should be a safe, easy, and inexpensive means of providing nutrition while waiting for the fistula to close. Some authors have also placed a double lumen gastrostomy tube with one lumen used to decompress the stomach, while the second lumen is passed into the jejunum through the gastrojejunostomy and used for alimentation purposes.[29] The aspirated material from the stomach may also be replaced into the jejunal tube, thereby avoiding the metabolic complications of prolonged gastric suction.

There have been three phases of fistula management described: (1) stabilization; (2) investigation; and (3) definitive therapy.[30] The stabilization phase consists of: (1) bowel rest and decompression; (2) histamine-2 (H_2)-blocker administration to decrease gastric output; (3) skin protection at the cutaneous site of the fistula to prevent the caustic action of the effluent; (4) ensure adequate drainage of the fistula; (5) ensure that all septic sites are controlled; (6) maintain fluid and electrolyte balance; and (7) provide adequate nutritional support.

The investigation phase does not commence until the fistula has been allowed to develop a good fibrous tract. This usually requires at least 1 week, and should be allowed to continue for at least 2 weeks to be sure a firm tract has formed. If the clinical condition of the patient deteriorates, the time schedule may be pushed up at the discretion of the attending physician. A fistulogram is the most useful test and will help define the anatomy of the fistula and determine if any conditions exist that contribute to fistula persistence. These include distal obstruction of the gastrointestinal tract, presence of abscesses, inadequate drainage of the fistula, or presence of a foreign body. The tract should be single without accompanying side tracts or loculations. Computed tomography may aid in the detection of intra-abdominal septic foci.

The definitive therapy phase is entered only if conservative therapy has failed to achieve closure of the fistula. Failure of medical management should not be considered until the fistula has persisted for at least 4 to 6 weeks. At that time, two courses may be taken. The fistula may be occluded or surgical intervention may be undertaken.

If during the investigation phase no reasons for fistula persistence are identified, the fistula may safely undergo a trial of closure by occlusion of the tract. A novel means of occluding the tract has been described by Jordan.[31] He blocks the external opening of the tract with a piece of bubble gum which has been chewed by the patient or made malleable by wetting and kneading. The gum is placed into the tract to occlude totally the entire length of the fistula and is held in place by a pressure dressing. He has reported excellent results with this technique with the prompt cessation of drainage and rapid healing.

In the unusual situation in which surgical takedown of the fistula becomes necessary, it is unwise to attempt closure of the duodenal opening via simple suture placement. These repairs frequently break down and sepsis or recurrent fistula results. The duodenal opening should be closed with a jejunal patch, just as described for the treatment of the initial wound.

Duodenal Obstruction

Obstruction of the intestinal lumen can occur wherever an anastomosis or suture line has been placed. This holds true for the duodenum as well. In addition, there are special problems that make obstruction in the duodenum a greater likelihood than in other portions of the bowel. The duodenum is a fixed retroperitoneal structure and adequate mobilization is difficult. The second portion is fixed to the pancreas and has a shared blood supply with the pancreas. The lumen of the duodenum may be small, making it more prone to obstruction from hematoma and edema. Edema of the duodenal wall may cause obstruction at the site of closure if the lumen has been significantly compromised by the repair. Also, edema in the head of the pancreas may cause obstruction of the duodenum.

At surgery, some of these causes can be anticipated and the surgery tailored to fit the clinical picture. If compromise of the lumen seems significant, one of the complex repairs should be performed. If pancreatic injury is apparent and significant edema is anticipated, then duodenal exclusion or diverticulization should be contemplated. Even the placement of a simple gastroenterostomy may avoid the postoperative problem.

If simple repair has been performed without any secondary protective procedure having been done, then it is mandatory that symptoms of duodenal obstruction be addressed. The initial method of management is to prolong the period of nasogastric suction. If symptoms do not resolve in about 10 days, then the duodenum should be evaluated via an upper gastrointestinal contrast study. After 10 days, the perioperative edema should have time to resolve and continued symptoms may herald a more serious cause for the obstruction. Nasogastric suction is continued for an additional week and the contrast study is then repeated. If the initial study demonstrated complete obstruction and there is no improvement on the 1 week follow-up study, then surgical intervention is indicated. When the initial study shows complete or partial obstruction and the follow-up study demonstrates marked improvement, then nasogastric suctioning is continued for another week and the study repeated. This course is continued until the duodenum opens up and the patient is symptom free, or progress stops, at which point surgical intervention is indicated.

When surgical intervention is required, it is preferable to perform a bypass procedure rather than trying to correct the obstruction at the point of the previous repair. Gaining adequate length for resection and reanastomosis will probably be almost impossible and the dissection will be very difficult due to the previous surgery and trauma. In the author's opinion it is preferable to perform a duodenojejunostomy or gastrojejunostomy, depending on the site of obstruction, rather than attempting a second repair, which will be fraught with danger.

INTRAMURAL DUODENAL HEMATOMA

This is a special and uncommon form of duodenal trauma found in victims of blunt abdominal trauma. Often, it is the only intra-abdominal injury present. The second and third portions of the duodenum are the most susceptible to this type of injury. The usual presenting symptoms are abdominal pain and bilious vomiting, which may not manifest themselves for several days after the trauma. Delays of 18 hours to 7 days have been reported.[32] The diagnosis is usually made via the upper gastrointestinal contrast study. This test not only will make the diagnosis, but also rule out perforation. The classic description is that of a coiled spring appearance of the duodenal mucosa with partial to complete obstruction.

In the past the form of therapy has been controversial, but recently a uniform therapeutic approach has been established. The majority of these injuries, particularly in children, will spontaneously resolve in 1 to 3 weeks.[33–35] Therefore the initial management is nasogastric suction with parenteral alimentation. Surgery is reserved for those patients who do not resolve with conservative therapy or have a demonstrated perforation. When surgery becomes necessary, it is usually possible to open the serosa and evacuate the hematoma. This easily relieves the source of obstruction. If local evacuation is not successful, then a bypass procedure should be considered. When a perforation is demonstrated, the surgical strategy is the same as for any duodenal disruption.

SUMMARY

Duodenal injuries are uncommon in the trauma patient, but when they occur they present unique challenges to the trauma surgeon. The potential for morbidity and mortality is high and is related to the severity of the duodenal defect, delay in diagnosis, adequacy of repair, and associated injuries. The latter factor has the most direct bearing on mortality.

It is essential that the surgeon maintain a high degree of suspicion in the patient with a mechanism of injury compatible with duodenal injury. The diagnosis must be aggressively pursued in the patient in whom a duodenal injury is suspected to avoid diagnostic delays. No laboratory test is diagnostic for duodenal injury, and the diagnosis must be made via radiographic studies.

Most injuries are amenable to repair by simple closure. The more severe injuries, as defined by established criteria, will require more complex reconstructive procedures. The type of repair should be tailored to the particular wound to ensure adequate debridement of devitalized tissue, and formation of a suture line without tension and with good blood supply. The best means to avoid the most common complication, a postoperative fistula, is to adhere to these principles. When a fistula does form, most may be managed medically with closure expected in 4 to 6 weeks. By adhering to the principle that the best defense is a good offense, treatment will result in acceptable morbidity and mortality rates in patients with duodenal trauma.

REFERENCES

1. Jordan GL: Injury to the pancreas and duodenum. In Mattox KL, Moore EE, Feliciano DV (eds): *Trauma*. Norwalk, CT: Appleton and Lange, 1988, pp 473–494.
2. Herzel M: Riss im Duodenum mit Villkommener drehung des Jejunums, Peritonitis, Laparotomie, Heilung. *Jahresber Chir* 1896;46:691.
3. Flint LM, McCoy M, Richardson JD, et al: Duodenal injury: Analysis of common misconceptions in diagnosis and treatment. *Ann Surg* 1980;191:697–702.
4. Ivatury RR, Nallathambi M, Gaudino J, et al: Penetrating duodenal injuries: Analysis of 100 consecutive cases. *Ann Surg* 1985;202:153–158.
5. Kelly G, Norton L, Moore G, et al: The continuing challenge of duodenal injuries. *J Trauma* 1978;18: 160–165.
6. Levison MA, Peterson SR, Sheldon GF, et al: Duodenal trauma: Experience of a trauma center. *J Trauma* 1984;24:475–480.
7. Stone HH, Fabian TC: Management of duodenal wounds. *J Trauma* 1979;19:334–339.
8. Snyder WH, Weigelt JA, Watkins WL, et al: The surgical management of duodenal trauma. Precepts based on a review of 247 cases. *Arch Surg* 1980;115:422–429.
9. Morton JR, Jordan GL: Traumatic duodenal injuries: Review of 131 cases. *J Trauma* 1968;8:127–139.
10. Bouwman DL, Weaver DW, Walt AJ: Serum amylase and its isoenzymes: A clarification of their implications in trauma. *J Trauma* 1984;24:573–578.

11. Greenlee T, Murphy K, Ram MD: Amylase isoenzymes in the evaluation of trauma patients. *Am Surg* 1984; 50:637–640.

12. Lucas CE, Ledgerwood AM: Factors influencing outcome after blunt duodenal injury. *J Trauma* 1975; 15:839–846.

13. Thal ER, McClelland RN, Shires GT: Abdominal trauma. In Shires GT (ed): *Principles of Trauma Care*. New York: McGraw-Hill Book Co., 1985, pp 291–344.

14. Cattel RB, Braasch JW: A technique for the exposure of the third and fourth portions of the duodenum. *Surg Gynecol Obstet* 1960;113:379–380.

15. Weigelt JA: Duodenal injuries. *Surg Clin North Am* 1990;70:529–539.

16. Cukingnan RA, Culliford AT, Worth MH: Surgical correction of a lateral duodenal fistula with the Roux-Y technique: Report of a case. *J Trauma* 1975;15:519–523.

17. DeShazo CV, Snyder WH, Daugherty CG, et al: Mucosal pedicle graft of jejunum for large gastroduodenal defects. *Am J Surg* 1972;124:671–672.

18. Kobold EE, Thal AP: A simple method for the management of experimental wounds of the duodenum. *Surg Gynecol Obstet* 1963;116:340–343.

19. Ivatury RR, Gaudino J, Ascer E, et al: Treatment of penetrating duodenal injuries: Primary repair vs. repair with decompressive enterostomy/serosal patch. *J Trauma* 1985;25:337–341.

20. McInnis WD, Aust JB, Cruz AB, et al: Traumatic injuries of the duodenum: A comparison of primary closure and the jejunal patch. *J Trauma* 1975;15:847–853.

21. Oreskovich MR, Carrico CJ: Pancreaticoduodenectomy for trauma: A viable option? *Am J Surg* 1984; 147:618–623.

22. Hasson JE, Stern D, Mass GS: Penetrating duodenal trauma. *J Trauma* 1984;24:471–474.

23. Berne CJ, Donovan AJ, White EJ, et al: Duodenal "diverticulization" for duodenal and pancreatic injury. *Am J Surg* 1974;127:503–507.

24. Vaughan GD, Frazier OH, Graham DY, et al: The use of pyloric exclusion in the management of severe duodenal injuries. *Am J Surg* 1977;134:785–790.

25. Martin TD, Feliciano DV, Mattox KL, et al: Severe duodenal injuries. Treatment with pyloric exclusion and gastrojejunostomy. *Arch Surg* 1983;118:631–635.

26. Kashuk JL, Moore EE, Cogbill TH: Management of the intermediate severity duodenal injury. *Surgery* 1982;92:758–764.

27. McKone TK, Bursch LR, Scholten DJ: Pancreaticoduodenectomy for trauma: A life-saving procedure. *Am Surg* 1988;54:361–364.

28. Heimansohn DA, Canal DF, McCarthy MC, et al: The role of pancreaticoduodenectomy in the management of traumatic injuries to the pancreas and duodenum. *Am Surg* 1990;56:511–514.

29. Lee SM: The use of double-lumen tubes in upper gastrointestinal surgery. *Am Surg* 1980;46:363–365.

30. Tarazi R, Coutsoftides T, Steiger E, et al: Gastric and duodenal cutaneous fistulas. *World J Surg* 1983;7: 463–473.

31. Jordan GL: Gastroenteric cutaneous fistula. *Arch Surg* 1964;88:540–546.

32. Touloukian RJ: Protocol for the nonoperative treatment of obstructing intramural duodenal hematoma during childhood. *Am J Surg* 1983;145:330–334.

33. Woolley MM, Mahour GH, Sloan T: Duodenal hematoma in infancy and childhood: Changing etiology and changing treatment. *Am J Surg* 1978;136:8–14.

34. Janson KL, Stokinger F: Duodenal hematoma: Critical analysis of recent treatment technics. *Am J Surg* 1975;129:304–308.

35. Jewett TC: Caldarola V, Karp MP, et al: Intramural hematoma of the duodenum. *Arch Surg* 1988;123:54–58.

8
Pancreas

NORMAN E. McSWAIN, JR., M.D., F.A.C.S.

The reported mortality rate from pancreatic trauma in the early part of the 1900s was 20–30%, with morbidity above 30%. The two most famous patients whose injuries were incompletely treated were President McKinley (1901) and President Garfield (1885). The circumstances that led to poor outcome relate to the retroperitoneal position of the gland, the difficulties in diagnosis, less than ideal anesthesia, lack of antibiotics, the caustic excretions of the gland, poor knowledge of the physiology and pathophysiology of resuscitation, and poor understanding of the technical methods of management. As surgeons gain more experience with trauma patients and their problems, the difficulties of injury to this gland will decrease. The postoperative abscess and fistula formation that followed treatment of pancreatic injuries made it an organ to be feared. Its anatomic position in close proximity to the duodenum, aorta, vena cava, portal venous system, splenic blood supply, colon, liver, and stomach signifies that associated injuries play a major role in the morbidity and mortality of pancreatic trauma.

President Garfield, for example, received a wound in the posterior abdomen.[1] Hemorrhage into the area from the splenic artery, lack of antibiotics, and lack of surgical experience with retroperitoneal abscesses led to incomplete drainage, sepsis, and subsequent blood loss that proved to be fatal some 6 weeks following the initial gunshot wound. Many patients today in trauma centers throughout the country survive similar injuries every night. President McKinley, on the other hand, lived only 8 days. The surgeons were more courageous, operating on him immediately, identifying the injury to the anterior and posterior stomach and affecting a repair with a "double row of fine black silk."[2] However, they were too timid to examine the retroperitoneum. Both the injury to the pancreas and to the kidney were missed. Eight days later, the President died of "gangrene of the stomach and pancreas" associated with probable intra-abdominal abscess caused by a *Staphylococcus*, electrolyte imbalance, hypovolemia, and generalized sepsis.[3] Today, on a nightly basis in trauma centers throughout the United States, these injuries are handled almost as a matter of routine with minimal mortality and morbidity. Better understanding of the anatomy and physiology of the retroperitoneum, especially the pancreas, antibiotics, intravenous fluids, and cardioactive medications provide the difference.

These various problems were evaluated in a review (1972–1979) from King-Drew Medical Center. Seven years experience with pancreatic trauma were analyzed.[4] The mortality and complications were directly related to the 2.1 other organs injured per patient. All the patients who died were in shock (<100 mm Hg systolic pressure) during the operative procedure, three died within 48 hours, the other three on day 9, 33, and 102. Since that time, improvements in blood replacement (safer blood and autotransfusion), transportation systems (improved prehospital care and more rapid hospital access), availability of trauma centers, improved diagnostic capabilities (computed tomography [CT] and endoscopic retrograde cholangiopancreatography [ERCP]), more experienced trauma surgeons, and improved operative techniques have lead to less mortality and morbidity.

An understanding of the problems of pancreatic injury is critical to the continued improvement in the outcome of these severe injuries.

ANATOMY

The pancreas is a complex organ anatomically, in addition to its retroperitoneal location. The splenic artery originates at the aorta and travels posterior to the pancreas along its upper border, providing blood supply to the body and tail of the organ while en route to the spleen (Fig. 8–1). At one, two, or even three areas along the cephalad border, a knuckle of the splenic artery will be visible above the superior margin of the pancreas. This positioning allows easy mobilization for distal pancreatectomy and secondary ligation after splenectomy. The body of the pancreas obtains its blood supply from an average of 7.6 branches of the splenic artery in its midportion and 5.3 branches in its distal third.[5] The arterial supply to the head of the pancreas comes from two (anterior and posterior) branches

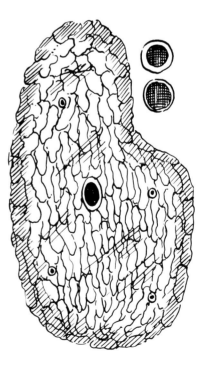

Figure 8–1. Splenic artery travels posterior to the pancreas and provides blood supply to the distal one half. Numerous anastomoses between the organ and the artery require ligation to preserve the spleen.

of the pancreatoduodenal artery. The superior component of both these arteries originates from the gastroduodenal artery as it becomes the right gastroepiploic artery. Both branches continue inferiorly on the anterior and posterior surface of the head of the pancreas to coalesce with the inferior pancreatoduodenal arteries that arise from the superior mesenteric artery. The anterior artery lies in the groove between the pancreas and the duodenum. The posterior branch of the artery is on the posterior surface of the gland. The head of the pancreas and duodenum (second and third portions) receives its blood supply from these vessels. Although both (anterior and posterior) have a dual source of origin, damage along the main length and subsequent interruption of local blood supply to either the pancreas or duodenum can produce ischemia to one or both organs. Injuries in the vicinity of this critical blood supply must be closely evaluated to decide if local repair or major resection (pancreatoduodenectomy) is the best approach.

The second concern in deciding whether the pancreas can be repaired is the status of the pancreatic duct. The main pancreatic duct begins at the tail of the pancreas. It courses the length of the gland near the center from cephalad to caudad, and just anterior to the midline in the anteroposterior (AP) direction. As the duct passes along the gland, branches join, just as creeks feed into a stream to make the stream a river. At or inside the head of the pancreas, this duct anastomoses with the common duct and courses to the duodenum to enter the lumen through the ampulla. The pancreatic duct may also enter into the lumen of the duodenum through a separate opening in the second portion.

The splenic vein runs along the posterior surface of the pancreas to anastomose with the superior mesenteric vein at approximately the junction between the middle third and head of the pancreas. This is just in the vicinity of the vertebral bodies. The vein lies caudad to the splenic artery and is approximately in the midposition of the pancreas. Venous drainage from the pancreas into the splenic vein averages, according to Dawson and Scott-Conner,[6] seven vessels in the distal third, 13 in the middle third, and six in the proximal third. These vessels are short, less than 2 mm in length. According to Skandalakis et al,[5] at least 13 vessels must be tied on the venous side to accomplish a distal pancreatectomy while preserving the spleen.

The uncinate process hooks caudad to the body and head of the pancreas to lie as a "J" resting on its side with the short portion of the "J" caudad. This caudad portion may empty into the duodenum via a separate duct or with the main duct.

The duodenum hooks around the head of the pancreas, beginning at the right lateral cephalad border, continuing around the head over the uncinate process, and along the caudad border. As would be expected from the name, the second and third portions of the duodenum and the head of the pancreas are supplied by the pancreaticoduodenal arteries. This combined blood supply renders resection of the head of the pancreas without the duodenum or the second and third portions of the duodenum without the head of the pancreas, difficult to impossible.

Pancreatic secretions are gathered from the acini by small ducts. These secretions flow toward the main pancreatic duct in ever enlarging arborizations. This main pancreatic duct, or canal of Wirsung, runs the length of the pancreas from the tail to the head. The duct usually empties into the duodenum along with the common duct at the ampulla of Vater. Secretions from the uncinate process empty via a smaller duct directly into the duodenum (duct of Santorini). These secretions can empty into the main pancreatic duct, as a common variant of the anatomic structure.

DIAGNOSIS

Diagnosis of pancreatic injuries is the most complicated component of the management of pancreatic trauma. The retroperitoneal location, lack of peritoneal covering, initial benign physical examination, and other factors make diagnosis of injuries to this organ by physical examination extremely difficult to almost impossible when the patient is initially seen after blunt injury. Delay in diagnosis, leading to repair more than 24 hours postinjury, significantly increases the morbidity and mortality rates.[6] The importance of early identification of pancreatic injury cannot be overemphasized. For example, Smith et al[7] reported a 237% increase in hospital days when pancreatic injury was not diagnosed in the first 24 hours following the traumatic incident. Attention to early and accurate diagnosis is important. The decision to operate on penetrating trauma is easy; the decision on blunt trauma is much more difficult.

History

As in the evaluation of any traumatic incident, the mechanism of injury is important in identifying the possible injuries that may be present.[8] A frontal impact in an automobile crash, incorrectly applied lap restraints, pedestrian impact from the front, handlebar injury from a motorcycle or bicycle, or other significant blunt trauma to the upper abdomen raises the possibility of pancreatic injury. The pancreas is trapped between the object external to the abdominal cavity in front and the vertebral column behind. Compression at this point can fracture the pancreas at the midpoint of the body or injure the duodenum in the fourth portion. Penetrating trauma of the upper abdomen can damage the head, body, or tail of the organ (Chapter 2).

Pain

Abdominal organs are insensitive to sensations other than stretch.[9] With mild to moderate pain or even pain enough to be readily noticed by the patient, inflammation must be present. The retroperitoneal location of the pancreas separates it from the peritoneum. Thus, the early indicators that identify inflammatory response by way of pain are no longer helpful. Pancreatic excretions must migrate from the injury point some distance to reach the peritoneal lining of the abdominal cavity. Pain therefore is not an early reliable sign. Even when present, the pain may be in the back, the epigastrium, or even in the shoulders. Other signs must be relied on to anticipate pancreatic injury.

Physical Examination

The symptoms of pancreatic damage, that is, the physical findings of direct tenderness, rebound tenderness, and muscular guarding, are late signs. Their absence cannot be used as a credible method to rule out pancreatic injury. Once these findings do develop, however, it must be assumed that there is significant inflammatory response already present. This inflammation will increase the complications and mortality rate. One should not await their presence to decide whether or not intervention is required.

A sudden decrease or absence of bowel sounds may be more helpful, since early inflammation often will diminish bowel activity before it will produce appreciable tenderness.

Laboratory

There is no laboratory evaluation technique that is particularly effective in diagnosing pancreatic injuries. The most discussed method is serum amylase. Jones[10] initially evaluated serum amylase and discovered that only 73% of patients with pancreatic injuries had an elevated amylase level. Patients with penetrating trauma were even less responsive (27%).[10] Olsen[11] found only 8% of patients with proven pancreatic injuries had an elevated serum amylase level. Stone et al[12] reported that 56% of patients with nonpenetrating trauma had an elevated amylase level. Bloch et al,[13] however, in studying acute alcoholism, identified 52% of patients with an overdose of alcohol had an elevated amylase greater than 300 IU/liter. Since the majority of patients had both blunt and penetrating trauma and had an elevated blood alcohol at presentation to the emergency room, it is extremely difficult to identify whether the source of the elevated amylase level is the alcoholic intake or if it truly represents pancreatic injury. Either way, it is not a valid test, especially since Moretz et al[14] reported that the majority of the amylase in acute alcoholism came from nonpancreatic sources. Such information makes a confusing picture as to the exact place, if any, that measurement of the serum amylase has in the recognition of pancreatic injuries following trauma. A rising amylase over several hours, on the other hand, probably does indicate that a pancreatic injury is present.

Computed Tomography

CT has been advocated by many as the ultimate test for evaluating retroperitoneal injuries.[15] A more complete discussion of the radiographic diagnostic techniques is found in Chapter 4. However, a group of investigators from San Francisco General Hospital (the originators of CT for evaluation of the bluntly traumatized patient) found, in a retrospective review of 300 patients with pancreatic trauma, that the CT scan only identified pancreatic injury correctly 73% of the time.[16] Of patients with significant injuries, including major ductal injuries, 15% were missed on CT obtained within the first 24 hours after trauma. A diagnosis of pancreatic injury made greater than 24 hours after the incident significantly increases the mortality rate; therefore, to rely on the CT as an evaluation method to rule out pancreatic injury is probably not sound. Other studies have reported similar results. Smith et al,[7] in reporting on 22 pediatric patients, identified that the CT was wrong 27% of the time when done early in the evaluation process. In the same study this group identified that patients with pancreatic injuries operated on within the first 24 hours, hospital stay was 16 days. Those who were diagnosed late had a significantly increased hospital stay of 38 days. Dodds et al[17] noted that the CT scan identified five pancreatic injuries but only four were found at time of surgery. Watanabe et al[18] looking at small bowel injuries found three false-negative examinations and two false-positive ones in 152 patients. Wisner et al[19] reviewed the results of the use of various techniques for the identification of small bowel injuries over a 39-month period. The CT was negative three of the four times that it was used. Although it might not seem that these studies relate, in fact, they are very important. One cannot rule out a pancreatic injury with a CT scan, while missing a bowel injury, and realistically expect the patient to do well. The trauma surgeon must be responsible for the entire patient. Other studies have reported both good and equivocal results with this technique. The present state-of-the-art of CT diagnosis is difficult at best and cannot be relied on for an accurate diagnosis unless the roentgenographer has extensive experience in analyzing CT studies of trauma. Even the most experienced may miss 15% of major injuries on a CT obtained early in the course of the developing pathology.

In reviewing the Charity Hospital experience in New Orleans, Frame et al[20] found a 20% incidence of missed injuries in CT scans interpreted by staff radiologists. In addition, many of the patients referred from other institutions for evaluation of head trauma had significant abdominal injuries that were missed by a faulty reading of a CT scan obtained prior to transfer.

Endoscopic Retrograde Cholangiopancreatography

The ERCP has been identified as a possible further diagnostic technique to be used in association with CT and physical examination in analyzing the presence or absence of ductal injury. Its use has been suggested as a diagnostic technique when all studies were normal but the kinematics of the incident indicated the possibility of pancreatic injury. Although the ERCP can be a useful adjunct, the patient must be placed in the prone position for an adequate pancreatogram. Such prone positioning of a patient with suspected or proven cervical, thoracic, or lumbar spine fractures is contraindicated. Patients with suspected spinal fractures or dislocations must undergo thorough evaluation of the spine for injury prior to ERCP. ERCP has been described for use in three different situations to evaluate pancreatic trauma.

Acute Evaluation

Patients with blunt abdominal trauma who had a high possibility of pancreatic injuries, but who had no obvious physical findings, were evaluated by Whittwell et al.[21] This small study was able to identify correctly patients with major ductal injury by using ERCP in patients who did not otherwise have proven pancreatic or other injuries. This method of evaluation is beneficial in those rare patients who have an isolated, pancreatic duct injury but no other intra-abdominal pathologic condition that will produce physical findings.

The accepted inaccuracy of the physical examination for the identification of pancreatic injuries early makes the utility of such a technique appealing. Long-term evaluation of the use of ERCP to determine its accuracy in the acute patient is necessary to identify, at the very least, the false-negative rate of the technique.

Intraoperative

Pancreatic injury without major ductal damage may not require diversion or partial resection, but only debridement and perhaps drainage. The correct diagnosis of ductal leakage may come from an intraoperative pancreatogram. Three methods of obtaining radiographic visualization of the pancreatic duct are via ERCP, transduodenal retrograde pancreatic duct catheterization, and catheter placement and pancreatogram in an antegrade fashion through the tail. LaRaja et al[22] reported on the use of intraoperative ERCP in 1986. Prior use had not been reported. A stab wound to the head of the pancreas was found to have produced an 8 cm hematoma. Although the pancreatic substance was injured anteriorly, posterior trauma was found. Intraoperative ERCP could identify no ductal leakage. No further treatment was instituted.

Since that time, similar reports have described limited usage of the technique. The questions of availability of an endoscope and an experienced endoscopist in the usual nocturnal trauma setting, time delay required for the procedure, and accuracy of the pancreatogram must be answered by the individual facility before it can be relied on as an oft used tool.

As was discovered with the initial hype following use of CT scan to evaluate blunt abdominal trauma, some institutions do it well, others do it not as well. One's own risk to benefit rate with ERCP must be evaluated before its use becomes routine within an institution and by a specific trauma team.

This test must be used judiciously, and by individuals skilled in its use in trauma. The exact role of this technique has not been defined.

Post-Trauma or Delayed

The patient who comes into the emergency department several days to weeks post-trauma with a suspicion of a pancreatic injury will benefit both from a CT scan and a ERCP. The CT scan can identify the presence of a pancreatic mass; however, the ERCP can assist the surgeon in deciding whether the patient requires operative intervention. Taxier et al[23] in 1980 reported the use of ERCP as a diagnostic tool in such patients. Six patients were seen 3 weeks to 6 years following blunt abdominal trauma. Five patients were demonstrated on ERCP to have ductal injury and underwent operative repair. The sixth patient had a normal ERCP. This patient was followed nonoperatively. No subsequent pancreatic problems were discovered. Hall et al[24] reported a similar experience in a small study of pediatric patients post-trauma. Two were evaluated early post-trauma and two were seen late.[24]

If one has the opinion, based on personal experience and case review, that a patient without pancreatic duct disruption should be treated nonoperatively, then ERCP represents an excellent diagnostic tool.

Ultrasound

As with the use of CT scan as a diagnostic tool to identify pancreatic injury, ultrasound may be a good tool also. Surgeons in the United States, however, do not have as much experience with this diagnostic device as do the Europeans. One report from the Hospital for Sick Children in Toronto describes the use of this tool in the evaluation of patients following blunt trauma to the abdomen.[25] Although one could certainly get into a lively discussion as to whether nonoperative management of patients who eventually developed pseudocysts was the correct approach, at least the ability of ultrasound to identify the pathologic condition has been demonstrated. Several of the patients in both groups were found to have "unexpected operative findings" that included pancreatic injury. The exact role that ultrasound played in missing the injuries was not presented. The reasons for nonoperative management of patients with obstructive pancreatitis and traumatic pseudocyst were not discussed. The authors did not describe the diagnostic accuracy of the ultrasound. However, they stated that it was "very helpful."

The usefulness of this technique in the diagnosis of pancreatic and other retroperitoneal injuries will require evaluation in several institutions before the exact role can be established.

Peritoneal Lavage

Analysis of the contents of the peritoneal cavity for blood, amylase, bacteria, and vegetable matter to determine retroperitoneal injuries of any type must be considered precarious. With the peritoneum intact, and in the absence of intra-abdominal injuries, logic would dictate that this test would be extremely inaccurate. It is!

MANAGEMENT

Several management techniques for pancreatic trauma have been developed. Observation, drainage, suture and drainage, distal pancreatectomy, Roux-en-Y pancreaticojejunostomy as a "living sucker," drain one or both halves of a midbody transection, or pancreatoduodenostomy and pancreatoduodenectomy (Whipple procedure) have all been proposed. Each is a good method of handling specific injuries. The management technique must be individualized to meet the peculiarities of the specific injury that exists. The only technique that has not been scientifically demonstrated to work, and that may produce more complications than it prevents, is drainage. Studies in draining other organ injuries, spleen and liver particularly, have an increased abscess rate.[26] Penrose and sump drains, or a combination of the two, are associated with hepatic abscesses in up to 25% of the patients managed in this manner.[27,28] Similar injuries when treated with no drain or with a closed suction drain have an abscess rate less than 5%. Sump versus closed drains were studied by Fabian et al.[79] Intra-abdominal abscess developed in 20% when sumps were used and only 2% when closed drainage was used.[29]

There are no data that demonstrate that patients with pancreatic injuries respond better with drains than without, although many authors suggest their use. Other authors have suggested in defense that they "do no harm." Stone et al[12] demonstrated that patients who had an open (Penrose) drain had a 46% abscess rate. Patients drained with a sump drain had only a 2% pancreatic complication rate.[12] This difference is important.

Distal Pancreatectomy

For injuries in the distal half of the pancreas, particularly when there is a major ductal injury, resection of the pancreas is usually the most appropriate procedure.

The technique for a distal pancreatectomy includes, as an essential component, closing the main pancreatic duct and minor ducts to prevent fistula formation. Hemostasis must also be obtained to prevent hematoma and the associated increased risks of abscess formation. Both can be achieved easily and quickly with a TA 90/TA 55 Linear stapler. Ligation of the duct and closing the capsule with either running or closely placed interrupted sutures to obtain a watertight closure is an alternate method.

Meticulous dissection is used to separate the pancreas from the splenic vein and artery. As identified in the "Anatomy" section, there are numerous vascular connections between the splenic vessels and the pancreas. The body and tail of the pancreas receive their major blood supply from these vessels. Dawson and Scott-Conner[6] and Skandalakis et al[5] in separate articles identified from 13 to 22 venous anastomoses that need to be controlled and seven to ten arterial anastomoses. These vessels are short, usually less than 1 to 2 mm in length outside the pancreatic capsule. Figure-of-eight vascular stitches directly in the vessel wall and a second figure-of-eight suture placed into the pancreatic capsule will most often produce the desired results.

The exact role for splenic preservation in trauma patients has not yet been defined. Prior to 1984, only one article in the literature identified overwhelming splenic sepsis in an adult when splenectomy was done after childhood. The long-term mortality and morbidity rate from adult postsplenectomy sepsis is less with splenectomy than the mortality and complication rate associated with the infusion of 4 units of banked blood.[26] There is no scientific justification for significant complex procedures, increased operative time, and increased transfusion rate to salvage the spleen. However, in patients with an isolated pancreatic injury, such meticulous dissection to preserve the splenic vasculature is probably justified if there is not an associated large blood loss producing the need for transfusions.

ROUX-EN-Y DRAINAGE PROCEDURES

As injuries approach nearer to the head of the pancreas, which if resected would require greater than 50% of the pancreas to be removed, the possibility of postoperative insulin deficiencies will be increased. This will also produce an increased possibility of damage to the portal vein. Some technique to preserve the pancreatic function of the tail following such trauma is justified. For pancreatic transection to the right of the vertebral column, or for injuries in this section that can be converted into a complete transection, Roux-en-Y drainage of the distal portion and oversewing or stapling of the proximal portion is a worthwhile technique (Fig. 8–2). This technique was first described by Letton and Wilson in 1959.[30] Because of the infrequent use of this technique, Laustsen et al[31] in 1988 reviewed the literature. They identified a total of 25 patients on whom this procedure had been attempted. Four minor and two major complications were noted. The complications and benefits of this technique have not been well documented in the literature.

For penetrating trauma, onlay of a "living sucker" sewn with a serosa-to-capsule technique onto the anterior surface of the pancreas provides excellent drainage anteriorly. The only difficulty is the posterior pancreatic surface. The defect, which one would certainly expect in the posterior pancreas, should be closed if possible. The "living sucker" can be wrapped around to include the defect on the posterior surface. Drainage only one component will not suffice. Resection of a small segment of the pancreas to make anastomosis with the "living sucker" more secure is possible.

As presented by Hendrickson and McSwain,[32] if the head of the pancreas and duodenum are injured in combination, especially by penetrating trauma, but the injury does

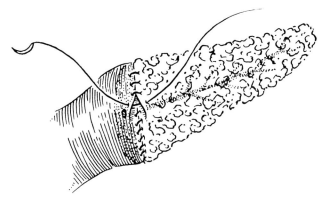

Figure 8–2.   Roux-en-Y drainage of the distal portion of the pancreas preserves the pancreatic secretions without running the risk of portal vein injury.

not compromise the blood supply, the posterior wound in the duodenum can be closed, and the anterior duodenum at the point of the injury can be reflected over the pancreatic injury (serosa to capsule, two layer). This will provide a secure closure (Fig. 8–3). Although patients who have an injury that can benefit from this procedure are few, its success demonstrates that with modification of existing accepted principles major resections can be avoided.

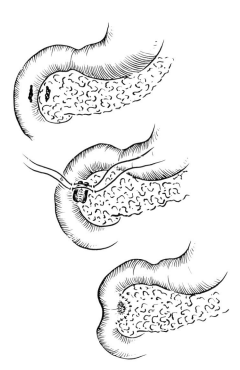

Figure 8–3.   Closure of the duodenum over an injured pancreas preserves function while protecting against leakage.

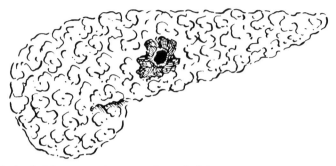

Figure 8–4.   The head of the pancreas is amputated near the injury.

Pancreatoduodenectomy

Severe injury to the head of the pancreas that compromises the blood supply or that produces significant damage to the duodenum will require a pancreatoduodenectomy. This procedure was first described by Whipple, for carcinoma of the ampulla, in 1935. The resection included the pancreatic head, the first, second, and third parts of the duodenum, and the distal common duct. Lowe et al[33] discussed its use in trauma in 1977.

The pancreatoduodenectomy is begun by a Kocher maneuver, mobilizing the duodenum and head of the pancreas to the vertebral column. The stomach is divided proximal to any injuries that may be present in the distal portion, up to a hemigastrectomy. If there is no injury to the stomach, the duodenum can be divided just distal to the pylorus. This will preserve the pyloric function. An equally acceptable approach is to use a hemigastrectomy. The jejunum and duodenum are separated just distal to the ligament of Treitz. The pancreas is cut as close to the injury as possible, taking care to preserve the superior mesenteric artery and portal vein (Fig. 8–4). The common duct is amputated through the cystic duct. This will allow a patch to be constructed to protect the choledochojejunal anastomosis (Fig. 8–5). The jejunum and head of the pancreas are then removed. The pancreaticojejunostomy is done in an end-to-end fashion. A choledochojejunostomy completes the right side of the hookup. The stomach is connected to the jejunum either at the duodenum, if a pyloric sparing anastomosis is desired, or a gastrojejunostomy, if not. All anastomoses are connected in a two-layer fashion, except for the choledochojejunostomy. This latter anastomosis is a single layer (Fig. 8–6).

One of the major complications associated with pancreatic resections is the anastomo-

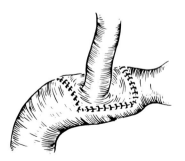

Figure 8–5.   Common duct is anastomosed to the jejunum in a patch fashion.

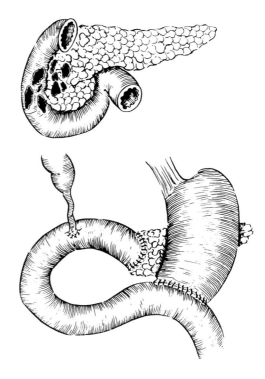

Figure 8–6. Completed operation.

sis of the pancreas to the small bowel. Another approach to this problem is not to attempt an anastomosis, but to ligate the duct. Gentilello et al[34] found that there was no difference in the morbidity and mortality between 13 patients so treated and that reported with the standard Whipple procedure. It must be pointed out, however, that most studies do not report a mortality rate of 53% with a Whipple procedure done for trauma.

MORBIDITY AND MORTALITY

Several reports in the literature of large enough series to be significant identify that the mortality rate of a pancreaticojejunostomy for trauma is in the range of 40%, although a recent small series had a 100% survival.[35] Pancreatic injuries, because of other associated injuries, have mortality rates exceeding 25%, but with an isolated pancreatic injury, the mortality rate is 5% or less. Stone et al[12] reported a 30-year experience from Grady Hospital. The overall mortality was 13.8%; the majority of this series was from penetrating injuries.

SUMMARY

Pancreatic injuries are difficult to diagnose due to their retroperitoneal location and lack of accurate diagnostic studies. Selection of diagnostic techniques must be tailored to the circumstances of each patient. Diagnosis that is delayed longer than 24 hours greatly increases the complication rate. When injuries are discovered, surgical approach must be individualized, utilizing one or a combination of several methods currently in use.

REFERENCES

1. Brooks SM (ed). *Our Assassinated Presidents: The True Medical Stories*. New York: Bell Publishing, 1985.
2. Ibid, p 152.
3. Ibid, p 165.
4. Sims EH, Mandal AK, Schlater T, Fleming AW, Lou MA: Factors affecting outcome in pancreatic trauma. *J Trauma* 1984;24:125–128.
5. Skandalakis JE, Gray SW, Rowe JS, Skandalakis LJ: Surgical anatomy of the pancreas. *Contemp Surg* 1979;14.
6. Dawson DL, Scott-Conner C: Distal pancreatectomy with splenic preservation: The anatomic basis for a meticulous operation. *J Trauma* 1986;26:1142–1145.
7. Smith SD, Nakayama DK, Gantt N, Lloyd D, Rowe MI: Pancreatic injuries in childhood due to blunt trauma. *J Pediatr Surg* 1988;23:610–614.
8. McSwain NE Jr: Mechanisms of injuries in blunt trauma. In McSwain NE Jr, Kerstein MD (eds): *Evaluation and Management of Trauma*. Norwalk, CT: Appleton-Century-Croft, 1987, pp 1–24.
9. Cope Z: *Cope's Early Diagnosis of the Acute Abdomen*, ed 17. Revised by William Silen. New York: Oxford University Press, 1987.
10. Jones RC: Management of pancreatic trauma. *Am J Surg* 1985;150:698–704.
11. Olsen WR: The serum amylase in blunt abdominal trauma. *J Trauma* 1973;13:200–204.
12. Stone HH, Fabian TC, Satiani MB, Turkleson ML: Experiences in the management of pancreatic trauma. *J Trauma* 1981;21:257–262.
13. Bloch RS, Weaver DW, Bouwman DL: Acute alcohol intoxication: Significance of the amylase level. *Ann Emerg Med* 1983;12:294–296.
14. Moretz JA III, Campbell DP, Parker DE, Williams GR: Significance of serum amylase level in evaluating pancreatic trauma. *Am J Surg* 1975;130:739–741.
15. Hauser CJ, Huprich JE, Bosco P, et al: Triple-contrast computed tomography in the evaluation of penetrating posterior abdominal injuries. *Arch Surg* 1987;122:1112–1115.
16. Jeffrey RB Jr, Federle MP, Crass RA: Computerized tomography of pancreatic trauma. *Radiology* 1983;147:491–494.
17. Dodds WJ, Taylor AJ, Erickson SJ, Lawson TL: Traumatic fracture of the pancreas: CT characteristics. *J Comput Assist Tomogr* 1990;14:375–378.
18. Watanabe S, Ishi T, Kamachi M, Takahashi T: Computed tomography and nonoperative treatment for blunt abdominal trauma. *Jpn J Surg* 1990;20:56–63.
19. Wisner DH, Chun Y, Blaisdell FW: Blunt intestinal injury. Keys to diagnosis and management. *Arch Surg* 1990;125:1322–1333.
20. Frame SB, Browder IW, Lang EK, McSwain NE: Computed tomography versus diagnostic peritoneal lavage: Usefulness in immediate diagnosis of blunt abdominal trauma. *Ann Emerg Med* 1989;18:513–516.
21. Whittwell AE, Gomez GA, Byers P, Kreis DJ Jr, Manten H, Casillas J: Blunt pancreatic trauma: Prospective evaluation of early endoscopic retrograde pancreatography. *South Med J* 1989;82:586–591.
22. LaRaja AD, Lobbato VJ, Cassaro S, Reddy RS: Intraoperative endoscopic retrograde cholangiopancreatography (ERCP) in penetrating trauma of the pancreas. *J Trauma* 1986;26:1146–1147.
23. Taxier M, Sivak MV Jr, Cooperman AM, Sullivan BH Jr: Endoscopic retrograde pancreatography in the evaluation of trauma to the pancreas. *Surg Gynecol Obstet* 1980;150:65–68.
24. Hall RI, Lavelle MI, Venables CW: Use of ERCP to identify the site of traumatic injuries of the main pancreatic duct in children. *Br J Surg* 1986;73:411–412.
25. Gorenstein A, O'Halpin D, Wesson DE, Daneman A, Filler RM: Blunt injury to the pancreas in children: Selective management based on ultrasound. *J Pediatr Surg* 1987;22:1110–1111.
26. Cerise EJ: Abdominal drains: Their role as a source of infection following splenectomy. *Ann Surg* 1970;171:764–769.
27. Noyes LD, Doyle DJ, McSwain NE Jr: Septic complications associated with the use of peritoneal drains in liver trauma. *J Trauma* 1988;28:337–346.
28. Gillmore D, McSwain NE Jr, Browder WI: Hepatic trauma: To drain or not to drain. *J Trauma* 1987;27:898–902.
29. Fabian TC, Kudsk KA, Croce MA, Payne LW, Mangiante EC, Voeller GR, Britt LG: Superiority of closed suction drainage for pancreatic trauma. A randomized, prospective study. *Ann Surg* 1990;211:724–730.

30. Letton AH, Wilson JP: Traumatic severance of pancreas treated by Roux-Y anastomosis. *Surg Gynecol Obstet* 1959;109:473–478.
31. Laustsen J, Jensen K, Bach-Nielsen P: Closed pancreatic transection treated by Roux-en-Y anastomosis. *Injury* 1988;19:42–43.
32. Henrickson M, McSwain NE Jr: Alternative method of managing head of pancreas injuries. Scientific exhibit, American College of Surgeons, 1988.
33. Lowe RJ, Saletta JD, Moss GS: Pancreatoduodenectomy for penetrating pancreatic trauma. *J Trauma* 1977;17:732–741.
34. Gentilello LM, Cortes V, Buechter KJ, Gomez GA, Castro M, Zeppa R: Whipple procedure for trauma: Is duct ligation a safe alternative to pancreaticojejunostomy? *J Trauma* 1991;31:661–667.
35. McKone TK, Bursch LR, Scholten DJ: Pancreaticoduodenectomy for trauma: A life-saving procedure. *Am Surg* 1988;54:361–364.

9

Extrahepatic Biliary Tract Injuries

GREGORY A. TIMBERLAKE, M.D., F.A.C.S.

Trauma to the extrahepatic biliary tract (which includes the hepatic ducts, the common bile duct, and the gallbladder and cystic duct) is uncommon. Failure to recognize injuries to the biliary tract, however, may result in significant morbidity and mortality for the patient. Additionally, improper management of an injury found at exploratory celiotomy for trauma may also result in an undesirable outcome with subsequent morbidity and possible mortality.

HISTORY

Little had been written about injuries to the extrahepatic biliary tree prior to the 19th century. Although wounds of the gallbladder undoubtedly were recognized before then, they were probably noted in association with wounds to the liver and other intra-abdominal structures, which resulted in death. During the Napoleonic Wars (1800–1815), Baron Larrey is said to have considered wounds of the gallbladder lethal because of the bile peritonitis that would result, even if other intra-abdominal injuries did not cause the patient's death. In 1799, Wainwright[1] published the first case report of a probable blunt rupture of the extrahepatic bile ducts. His patient had fallen from a horse and, after an initial period of "shock," developed abdominal distention, jaundice, and inanition ultimately resulting in death 8 weeks later. At autopsy, he was found to have 12 to 15 liters of bilious ascites with an intact gallbladder and a dilated hepatic duct. No actual communication to the biliary tree was demonstrated, however. Several years later, Fizeau[2] reported on a case of bile duct rupture in the French literature and described the symptoms of rupture of the common bile duct due to blunt trauma.

The first report in the English language was by Drysdale in 1861.[3] A 13-year-old boy sustained blunt trauma to the abdomen and subsequently developed a bile-containing "cyst" of the abdomen, which was drained 21 days after injury. However, he ultimately succumbed some 53 days after injury. Battle,[4] in 1894, is given credit for the next description of common bile duct transection due to blunt abdominal trauma. His report describes the case of a 6-year-old boy with blunt trauma causing common bile duct rupture who had drainage of his bilious ascites 7 days after injury but died the next day.

110

It was not until 1939 that Lysaght[5] described the first survivor from common bile duct transection: an 82-year-old man who had his injury diagnosed within 24 hours and underwent ligation of the proximal common duct and cholecystogastrostomy. The patient was doing well when last seen 3 months after his operation.

Brown[6] in 1932 reported the first case of traumatic cholecystectomy in which the gallbladder had been completely ripped free from the gallbladder fossa. Since that time, there have been more and more frequent reports published in the literature and there are now well over 500 reports of biliary tract injuries from external trauma.

ANATOMY

The extrahepatic biliary tract (Fig. 9–1) consists of the hepatic duct (also known as the excretory duct of the liver), the gallbladder (and the cystic duct, which is the continuation of the gallbladder), and the common bile duct. The common bile duct is formed by the union of the hepatic and cystic ducts. These structures run in the hepatoduodenal ligament with the portal vein and the hepatic artery and its branches. Lying ventrally are the bile ducts and the hepatic artery, with the bile ducts in the lateral free edge of the hepatoduodenal ligament. Dorsal to these structures lies the portal vein.

The hepatic duct is formed in the hilum of the liver, in the depths of the transverse fissure, by the union of the right and left hepatic ducts. The resulting duct runs inferiorly, posteriorly, and medially in the gastrohepatic ligament. The length of this duct varies

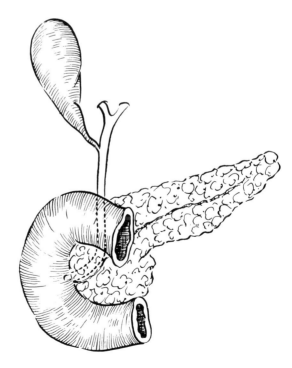

Figure 9–1. Schematic illustrations of the gross anatomy of the extrahepatic biliary tract.

considerably but averages 4 cm. The length of the duct depends on the level at which it is joined by the cystic duct. In the liver hilum the hepatic duct crosses the portal vein and the hepatic artery's branches. As the duct leaves the hilum, it lies over the anterolateral aspect of the portal vein, a relationship that it maintains to its termination. The cystic artery, usually arising from the right hepatic artery, runs posterior to the hepatic duct and then ramifies over the anterior surface of the neck of the gallbladder. The cystic artery may divide into distinct anterior and posterior branches as it reaches the gallbladder.

The gallbladder is a thin-walled, pear-shaped reservoir for the accumulation and concentration of bile. With a capacity of about 50 cc it is 8 to 10 cm long. It is attached to the liver by loose connective tissue and by peritoneum reflecting from its sides. The fundus of the gallbladder, a large bulbous structure, is partly covered by peritoneum and occupies the cystic notch in the margin of the liver and extends past it for a distance of at least 1.0 cm. When full, the gallbladder fundus may come into contact with the anterior abdominal wall opposite the ninth costal margin. The body of the gallbladder lies against the inferior surface of the liver. Normally, the body of the gallbladder is attached to the liver fossa with no intervening peritoneum. Rarely, the gallbladder may be attached quite loosely, be freely mobile, and appear to be suspended from the liver by a mesentary. Of note, small vessels and small accessory biliary ducts (of Luschka) may run directly from the liver to the gallbladder. The surgical significance of the ducts of Luschka is that failure to recognize them may result in injury to these ducts during cholecystectomy; if transected, these ducts should be ligated when recognized.[7] If not ligated, they may lead to a postoperative bile leak. The body of the gallbladder then tapers into the neck, which has a sinuous course to its termination in the cystic duct. The neck of the gallbladder is found in the uppermost free portion of the lesser omentum and contains the remnants of the embryonic spiral valves of Heister. In the neck, between the body and the cystic duct, may be found an anterior bulge known as the ampulla.

The medial continuation of the neck of the gallbladder becomes the cystic duct. This duct is up to 4 cm in length but is often so folded upon itself that its junction with the hepatic duct may appear quite close to the neck of the gallbladder. The cystic duct may run some distance parallel to the hepatic duct before opening into it. Many variations of the junction of cystic duct with the hepatic duct are found in man. The cystic duct contains a series of folds of redundant mucosa called the spiral valves of Heister. Running along with the cystic duct, usually on its left side, is the cystic artery.

The common bile duct is the direct continuation of the hepatic duct after the junction of the cystic and hepatic ducts. Usually about 9 cm long, it may be thought of as having four portions: the supraduodenal portion, running in the lesser omentum; the retroduodenal portion, lying behind the duodenum; the pancreatic portion, lying in a groove in or behind the pancreas; and an intraduodenal portion, descending obliquely through the duodenum. Many anomalies of the common bile duct have been described in man. These anomalies are of great importance to the surgeon and the reader is referred to standard anatomy texts for further details.

The first portion of the duct is about 3.5 cm long. This supraduodenal portion descends along the right or free margin of the lesser omentum on the right of the hepatic artery and anterior to the portal vein. The second portion of the duct runs behind the first part of the duodenum, to the right of the portal vein, and anterior to the vena cava. The third, or pancreatic, portion of the duct runs along the posterior surface of the pancreas, either in the substance of the gland or in a pancreatic groove. This portion of the duct ends by piercing the posterior medial aspect of the second part of the duodenum. It is separated from the inferior vena cava by a thin layer of pancreas or by connective tissue alone. The portal vein has no direct relationship to this portion of the duct, but on its left side the gastroduodenal artery is adjacent to the duct. The common duct is crossed either anteriorly or posteriorly by a branch of this artery, the superior pancreaticoduodenal trunk. The final, or intraduodenal, portion of the duct begins as the pancreatic portion enters the duodenal wall obliquely. The distal common bile duct is usually joined on its left by the pancreatic duct. Distally, there is a short common reservoir formed by these two ducts known as the ampulla of Vater. This structure becomes constricted and then opens into the duodenum at the duodenal papilla. The caliber of the common bile duct begins to taper as soon as it enters the duodenum.

An extremely important concept for the trauma surgeon is that of the vascular supply of the common bile duct (Fig. 9–2). The common bile duct is a very vascular structure, especially in its retroduodenal portion. There is a rich epicholedochal arterial plexus sheathing the common bile duct. This plexus is primarily derived from the posterosuperior pancreaticoduodenal artery, although considerable variation in the origin of this blood supply exists. A rich intramural arterial plexus is also present and is very important in surgical management of common bile duct injuries. The classic anatomic description of the blood supply of the common duct is by Parke et al.[8] Proximally, the epicholedochal

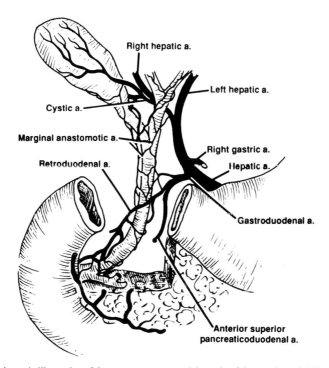

Figure 9–2.   Schematic illustration of the most common arterial supply of the extrahepatic biliary tract. Note the multiple anastomosis with surrounding arteries and the importance of the medial and lateral marginal anastomotic vessels to the blood supply of the supraduodenal portion of the common bile duct. For clarity, the retroportal artery is not shown.

plexus receives contributions from the hepatic and cystic arteries. The recently described retroportal artery provides an important source of collateral blood supply to the supra-duodenal portion of the common bile duct.[9] Depending on its route and distal connections, the retroportal artery supplies the supraduodenal portion from below in only two thirds of patients and from above in one third of patients.[10] Despite this generous blood supply, stripping the adventitia and denuding the common bile duct may damage the longitudinal arteries running along the side of the supraduodenal portion and may result in an avascular stricture. This propensity for stricture formation may explain why primary repairs of complex injuries of the supraduodenal common bile duct fare so poorly.

CLINICAL MANAGEMENT OF EXTRAHEPATIC BILIARY TRACT INJURIES

Injuries to the extrahepatic biliary tract from external violence are uncommon. The over-all incidence is only 3 to 5% in all abdominal trauma victims. Most of these are injuries to the gallbladder and the most common etiology is penetrating trauma (Table 9–1). Blunt injury to the gallbladder is less common and blunt injury to the bile ducts is rare, although perhaps increasing in our modern, high-speed society. Associated intraperitoneal injuries are frequent, with injury to the liver or the major intra-abdominal blood vessels being the most common (Table 9–2). In the majority of cases, the associated injuries determine the patient's clinical presentation, surgical treatment, and ultimate outcome.[11–15]

Preoperative diagnosis of an extrahepatic biliary tract injury is often very difficult. Bile may not be found on peritoneal lavage even when a biliary tract injury is present, but even if bile is found, its presence is not specific and the source may be the liver or the small bowel.

When the patient has other indications for celiotomy, the presence of blood or bile in the subhepatic space suggests injuries to the hepatoduodenal ligament structures and mandates thorough exploration of the portal vein, extrahepatic bile ducts, and gallbladder. Injury to the hepatic artery or portal vein should be controlled first, as described in the chapter on the diagnosis and treatment of these injuries. If bile has been found, but no obvious injuries to the bile ducts or gallbladder have been seen, then intraoperative cholangiography should be performed in an attempt to define the area of injury.

During celiotomy for blunt abdominal trauma, the presence of a small amount of bile in the subhepatic space may be difficult to visualize. A technique that may be useful, after initial exploration of the subhepatic space (which must include mobilization of the duodenum with a Kocher maneuver and inspection of the entire extrahepatic biliary system), is to place a clean dry radiopaque sponge in the subhepatic space. After the rest of the abdomen has been reexplored, the sponge is examined for the presence of any bile. Bile staining of the sponge in the absence of an obvious injury to the biliary tract is another indication for intraoperative cholangiography.

Isolated injury to the extrahepatic biliary tract is rare. Signs and symptoms are characteristically slow to appear in the absence of associated injuries. Initially, the uncontaminated and uninfected bile which has spilled does not cause chemical irritation to the peritoneum and peritoneal signs may be lacking. Even the abdominal pain from leakage of concentrated bile secondary to injury to the gallbladder may abate after a few hours of observation. If unrecognized, these injuries may lead to death. Means[16] reported an

Table 9–1   Spectrum of Injuries to the Extrahepatic Biliary Tract

REFERENCE	GB AND/OR CD*		HD AND/OR CBD*		GB AND DUCTAL*		TOTAL	
	PENETRATING	BLUNT	PENETRATING	BLUNT	PENETRATING	BLUNT	PENETRATING	BLUNT
Kitahama et al[11]	25	4	6	1	3	1	34	6
Posner and Moore[12]	25	7	5	0	0	0	30	7
Ivatury et al[13]	33	5	10	0	1	1	44	6
Bade et al[14]	44	1	4	4	0	0	48	5
Total	127	17	25	5	4	2	156 (87%)	24 (13%)
	80%		17%		3%		100%	

*GB: gallbladder; CD: cystic duct; HD: hepatic duct; CBD: common bile duct.

**Table 9–2   Associated Organ Injuries in 211 Patients
with Extrahepatic Biliary Tract Injuries**

ORGAN INJURED	KITAHAMA ET AL[11]	POSNER ET AL[12]	IVATURY ET AL[13]	BADE ET AL[14]	SODERSTROM ET AL[40]	TOTAL (% PATIENTS)
Liver	33	27	39	35	25	159 (75)
Major vascular	15	7	14	7	14	57 (27)
Duodenum	9	7	14	5	0	35 (17)
Pancreas	7	3	9	4	6	29 (14)
Stomach	14	3	4	5	0	26 (12)
Colon	7	9	3	6	0	25 (12)
Urologic	8	5	7	3	1	24 (11)
Small bowel	4	0	4	6	9	23 (11)
Spleen	3	2	2	0	11	18 (9)
Diaphragm	0	2	3	8	3	16 (8)
None	3	0	0	6	1	10 (5)
Total	103	65	99	85	70	422

85% mortality in his group of patients with bile peritonitis. The mortality if bile peritonitis develops remains as high as 30% even today.[17] Despite this, the clinical course of such patients may be surprisingly prolonged and the diagnosis of extrahepatic biliary tract injury delayed for hours, days, or even weeks.[18–20] Patients have been discharged from the hospital only to return with infected bile peritonitis or clinical pictures simulating ampullary carcinoma with weight loss and obstructive jaundice.[18,19,21–23] The patient's symptoms can be particularly perplexing if biliary tract injury was not recognized at laparotomy. When there has been a delay in the initial diagnosis of a patient's extrahepatic biliary tract injury, many ancillary tests may be useful to identify and define the extent of injury. These include abdominal computed tomography scanning, radionucleutide hepatobiliary scanning, abdominal ultrasonography, endoscopic retrograde cholangiopancreatography, and percutaneous transhepatic cholangiography.[22–27]

INJURIES TO THE EXTRAHEPATIC BILE DUCTS

Bile duct injuries are usually classified as either simple or complex.[28,29] Simple injuries are those defined as having tangential lacerations that involve less than 50% of the duct wall circumference. Complex injuries by definition are those with lacerations involving more than 50% of the duct wall circumference, segmental loss of a portion of the duct wall or complete ductal transection.

With penetrating trauma, the common bile duct is more commonly injured than the hepatic duct. The right hepatic duct is more often injured then the left hepatic duct. With blunt trauma, disruption of the common bile duct at the pancreaticoduodenal junction is usual.[30] The mechanism of injury is thought most likely to be a deceleration or compression of the right upper quadrant of the abdomen, suddenly moving the liver cephalad, causing a tear of the common bile duct at the junction of the supraduodenal and retroduodenal portions. At this point, the duct is fixed to the pancreas.[30,31]

Once the extent of injury has been determined and the associated injuries have been dealt with, the method for repair of the extrahepatic bile duct injuries is chosen, primarily dependent on the overall condition of the patient. If the patient is hemodynamically unstable, then splinting of the damaged duct with a T-tube and external drainage with planned staged repair may be the most appropriate initial treatment. The surgeon must remember that external drainage alone is seldom successful as definitive treatment.[32] If biliary fistula, intraperitoneal bile collection, or sepsis supervene in the immediate postoperative period, then the patient often must undergo reoperation in a surgical field complicated by the presence of inflammation and adhesions, thus making secondary procedures much more difficult.

If the patient is hemodynamically stable, has no severe underlying cirrhosis, or a coagulopathy, then definitive repair of the ductal injury may be performed. For simple injuries of the bile duct (by definition involving less than the 50% of the ductal wall diameter), definitive treatment consists of primary suture repair of the injury, T-tube placement through a separate incision, and external drainage. The presence of the T-tube serves to decompress the biliary tree in the early postoperative period when edema may obstruct or limit drainage to the distal common bile duct. The presence of the T-tube also will allow for postoperative cholangiography.

For complex ductal injuries, primary suture repair or primary reanastomosis should be avoided because the long-term stricture rate is over 50%.[13,33–35] Biliary stricture, which is the major late morbidity from bile duct trauma, almost always necessitates reoperation to prevent recurrent cholangitis or biliary cirrhosis. The vascular anatomy of the common bile duct, discussed earlier, may help explain the high stricture rate after primary repairs of complex injuries.[8–10]

If the patient has a bile duct injury with laceration involving more than 50% of the ductal wall circumference, segmental loss of a portion of the ductal wall, or a complete transection, then the treatment of choice is construction of a biliary-enteric anastomosis and external drainage.[11–13,29,34,35] The biliary-enteric anastomosis chosen will be dictated by anatomic considerations found at surgery. If the complex injury is found to involve the common hepatic duct or the right or left hepatic duct, then hepaticojejunostomy with cholecystectomy and external drainage is the best treatment. For complex common bile duct injuries, a choledochojejunostomy is the treatment of choice. To minimize enteric leaks in both cases, a defunctionalized loop of jejunum should be used. Either a Roux-en-Y or a simple jejunal loop with a distal enteroenterostomy may be used when constructing either the hepaticojejunostomy or choledochojejunostomy. In either case, the anastomosis should be performed with a single layer of fine suture. We prefer 5-0 or 6-0 polypropylene suture, although polygalactin or other monofilament suture will probably work as well. Whatever suture is used, mucosa to mucosa approximation must be achieved.

With either hepaticojejunostomy or choledochojejunostomy, the late stricture rate has reported to be only about 5% in complex bile duct injuries.[13,34,35]

Choledochoduodenostomy cannot be recommended in traumatic wounds of the bile ducts because of the possibility of anastomotic leak, which then develops into a lateral duodenal fistula. The complications from this are much more serious than a leak from a defunctionalized loop of jejunum. Additionally, it may be technically quite difficult to perform a choledochoduodenostomy when the patient has a normal- or small-sized common bile duct.

Cholecystojejunostomy with ligation of the injured common bile duct is also not recommended. As described earlier, the cystic duct may run parallel and even share a common wall with the common hepatic duct for a variable distance. The danger exists than an intramural cystic duct may be ligated along with the distal "common" duct, thus creating a nonfunctional anastomosis. This problem unfortunately would not be recognized until the development of postoperative jaundice. Also, long-term patency of the cystic duct cannot be guaranteed.

As with any traumatic injury, meticulous attention to the details of surgical technique is essential. Failure to follow these guidelines may result in fistulas and late stricture formation. Nonviable tissue must be debrided. The area of injury must be meticulously dissected. Any reconstruction performed must be made without tension and have a mucosa to mucosa approximation. The surgeon must keep the anatomy of the blood supply of the bile ducts in mind while mobilizing the common bile duct to avoid accidental injuries to the blood supply of the duct, which may result in late bile duct stricture from ischemia.

In all repairs of the extrahepatic bile ducts, external drainage using a closed suction drainage catheter should be instituted. The drain should be placed through a separate stab incision. Such drainage is important not only to control any leakage from the biliary tract repairs but to drain any bile leakage if an accessory duct of Luschka has been damaged.[7]

INJURIES TO THE GALLBLADDER

Injuries to the gallbladder and cystic duct remain the most common types of extrahepatic biliary tract trauma. The vast majority of such injuries are penetrating, although blunt injuries are being reported with increasing frequency.

A useful classification scheme for gallbladder injuries divides them into four categories.[36,37] The first is rupture (or perforation or laceration) which is the most common gallbladder injury. Avulsion, the second category, usually results from rapid deceleration injuries with shearing forces that tear the fluid-filled gallbladder from the liver bed. The avulsion may be partial or complete. If complete, the gallbladder may be found hanging by its attachment to the cystic duct and artery. The third category is contusion. Blunt trauma, usually from direct compression, may result in ecchymosis of the gallbladder wall only. Mild contusions may spontaneously resolve, but intramural hematoma from the contusion may result in ischemic necrosis of that segment of the gallbladder wall with subsequent delayed rupture of the gallbladder. The fourth category is acalculous cholecystitis purportedly from hemobilia resulting in blood in the gallbladder. Blood clots may then block the cystic duct and result in acute cholecystitis. A very rare form of gallbladder injury is traumatic biliary peritonitis without perforation, thought to result when the mucosal lining of the gallbladder has been disrupted.[38]

The treatment of gallbladder injuries is predicated on the hemodynamic stability of the patient. If the patient is hemodynamically stable, then cholecystectomy is the preferred treatment for any gallbladder injury with the possible exception of the most minor gallbladder wall contusion.

Cholecystorrhaphy has been used successfully and advocated to treat patients with penetrating gallbladder trauma.[14,36,39] It has the theoretical risk of gallstone formation because of sutures placed in the gallbladder wall and the risk of bile leakage from the suture line. Because of these problems, cholecystorrhaphy is not advocated as the treatment of choice today, at least in adult patients. The role of cholecystorrhaphy in pediatric gallbladder trauma remains to be defined.

Cholecystostomy is another option that has been used successfully. It may be particularly useful in the multiply traumatized patient who has developed a severe coagulopathy or has underlying cirrhosis. It may also be used in the hemodynamically unstable patient with severe associated injuries and minor damage to the gallbladder. One serious concern with the use of cholecystostomy in trauma patients is its reported high incidence of biliary fistula formation.[14]

As mentioned earlier, some minor gallbladder injuries, specifically contusions, may resolve without the need for surgical intervention. If there is any question of the extent of injury, however, then cholecystectomy should be considered.[40,41]

After any of these surgical procedures has been performed, a closed suction drain should be placed into the subhepatic space through a separate stab wound. This drain will also serve to control any bile leakage if an accessory duct of Luschka has been damaged either by the original trauma or the surgical procedure.[7]

SUMMARY

Extrahepatic biliary tract injuries, while infrequent, have significant morbidity and mortality associated with them if the injuries are either initially missed or if a primary repair of a complex ductal injury is attempted. The mortality seen with extrahepatic biliary tract trauma is in most cases related to the morbidity and mortality from associated organ system injuries. Major intra-abdominal vascular and neurologic injuries account for the majority of deaths.

Proper management of these injuries depends on a high index of suspicion during the initial evaluation and celiotomy. If gallbladder injury is found, then the treatment of choice is cholecystectomy. For simple injuries of the bile ducts, primary suture repair with T-tube placement and external drainage often suffices. For complex bile duct injuries, a biliary-enteric anastomosis is the preferred treatment, again with external drainage. Lesser procedures than these should be reserved for the hemodynamically unstable patient, the patient who has developed a severe coagulopathy, or who has severe underlying cirrhosis. In these latter patients, plans should be made at the time of initial surgery for a secondary reconstruction.

REFERENCES

1. Wainwright T: (Letter). *Med Phys J (Lond)* 1799;362–364.
2. Fizeau L: Observation sur une rupture du conduit choledoque avec epanchement dans le ventre, suivie d'autres observations analogues a des reflections sur la couleur jaune des icteriques. *J Med Chir Pharmcol* 1806;12:171.
3. Drysdale TM: Case of rupture of the common duct of the liver. Formation of a cyst containing bile. Death occurring on the fifty third day. Autopsy. *Am J Med Sci* 1861;12:399–404.
4. Battle WH: Traumatic rupture of the common bile duct. *Trans Clin Soc Lond* 1894;27:144–148.
5. Lysaght AD: A case of traumatic severance of the common bile duct. *Br J Surg* 1939;26:646.
6. Brown HPJ: Traumatic cholecystectomy. *Ann Surg* 1932;95:952–953.
7. McQuillan T, Manolas SG, Hayman JA, Kune GA: Surgical significance of the bile duct of Luschka. *Br J Surg* 1989;76:696–698.
8. Parke WW, Michels NA, Ghosh GM: Blood supply of the common bile duct. *Surg Gynecol Obstet* 1963;117:47–55.
9. Northover JMA, Terblanche J: Bile duct blood supply: Its importance in human liver transplantation. *Transplantation* 1978;26:67–69.

10. Northover JMA, Terblanche J: A new look at the arterial supply of the bile duct in man and its surgical implications. *Br J Surg* 1979;66:379–384.
11. Kitahama A, Elliott LF, Overby JL, Webb WR: The extrahepatic biliary tract injury: Perspectives in diagnosis and treatment. *Ann Surg* 1982;196:536–540.
12. Posner MC, Moore EE: Extra-hepatic biliary tract injury: Operative management plan. *J Trauma* 1985;25:833–837.
13. Ivatury RR, Rohman M, Nallathambi M, Rao PM, Gunduz Y, Stahl WM: The morbidity of injuries of the extra-hepatic biliary system. *J Trauma* 1985;25:967–973.
14. Bade PG, Thomsom SR, Hirshberg A, Robbs JV: Surgical options in traumatic injury to the extrahepatic biliary tract. *Br J Surg* 1989;75:256–258.
15. Dawson DL, Johansen KH, Jurkovich GJ: Injuries to the portal triad. *Am J Surg* 1991;161:545–551.
16. Means RL: Bile peritonitis. *Am Surg* 1964;30:583–588.
17. Ackerman NB, Sillin LF, Suresh K: Consequences of intraperitoneal bile: Bile ascites versus bile peritonitis. *Am J Surg* 1985;149:244–246.
18. Hartman SW, Greaney EM: Traumatic injuries to the biliary system in children. *Am J Surg* 1964;108: 150–156.
19. Zollinger RM Jr, Keller RT, Hubay CA: Traumatic rupture of the right and left hepatic ducts. *J Trauma* 1972;12:563–569.
20. Michelassi F, Ranson JHC: Bile duct disruption by blunt trauma. *J Trauma* 1985;25:454–457.
21. Abou-Mourad NN, Rogers LS: Extrahepatic biliary steering-wheel trauma simulating pancreatic carcinoma. *J Trauma* 1980;20:180–182.
22. Burt TB, Nelsom JA: Extrahepatic biliary duct trauma: A spectrum of injuries. *West J Med* 1981;134: 283–289.
23. Gately JG, Thomas EJ: Post-traumatic ischemic necrosis of the common bile duct. *Can J Surg* 1985;28: 32–33.
24. Frank DJ, Pereiras R, Souza-Lima MD, Taub SJ, Schiff ER: Traumatic rupture of the gallbladder with massive biliary ascites. *JAMA* 1987;240:252–253.
25. Spigos DG, Tan WS, Larson G, Palani C, Zaitoon MM, Capek V: Diagnosis of traumatic rupture of the gallbladder. *Am J Surg* 1981;141:731–735.
26. Gottesman L, Marks RA, Kloury PT, Moallem AG, Wichern WA Jr: Diagnosis of isolated perforation of the gallbladder following blunt trauma using sonography and CT scan. *J Trauma* 1984;24:280–281.
27. Jones KB, Thomas E: Traumatic rupture of the hepatic duct demonstrated by endoscopic retrograde cholangiography. *J Trauma* 1985;25:445–449.
28. Feliciano NV, Bitondo CG, Burch JM, Mattox KL, Beall AC Jr, Jordan GL Jr: Management of traumatic injuries to the extrahepatic biliary ducts. *Am J Surg* 1985;150:705–709.
29. Pachter HL, Liang HG, Hofstetter SR: Injury to the liver and biliary tract. In Mattox KL, Moore EE, Feliciano DV (eds): *Trauma.* Norwalk CT: Appleton and Lange, 1988, pp 429–442.
30. Fletcher WS, Mahnke DE, Dunphy JE: Complete division of the common bile duct due to blunt trauma. Report of a case and review of the literature. *J Trauma* 1961;1:87–95.
31. Fish JC, Johnson GL: Rupture of duodenum following blunt trauma: Report of a case with avulsion of papilla of Vater. *Ann Surg* 1965;162:917–919.
32. Carmichael DH: Avulsion of the common bile duct by blunt trauma. *South Med J* 1980;73:166–168.
33. Lee JG, Wherry DC: Traumatic rupture of the extrahepatic biliary duct from external trauma. *J Trauma* 1961;1:105–114.
34. Busuttil NW, Kitahama A, Cerise E, McFadden M, Lo R, Longmire WP Jr: Management of blunt and penetrating injuries to the porta hepatis. *Ann Surg* 1980;191:641–648.
35. Sheldon GF, Lim RC, Yee ES, Peterson SR: Management of injuries to the porta hepatis. *Ann Surg* 1985;202:539–545.
36. Smith SW, Hastings TN: Traumatic rupture of the gallbladder. *Ann Surg* 1954;139:517–520.
37. Pen I: Injuries to the gallbladder. *Br J Surg* 1962;49:636–641.
38. Solheim K: Blunt gallbladder injury. *Injury* 1972;3:246–248.
39. Hall ER Jr, Howard JM, Jordan GL, Mikesky WE: Traumatic injuries of the gallbladder. *Arch Surg* 1956;72:520–524.
40. Soderstrom CA, Maekawa K, DuPriest RW Jr, Cowley RA: Gallbladder injuries resulting from blunt abdominal trauma. *Ann Surg* 1981;193:60–66.
41. McNabney WK, Rudek R, Pemberton LB: The significance of gallbladder trauma. *J Emerg Med* 1990;8:277–280.

10

Colon

NORMAN E. McSWAIN, JR., M.D., F.A.C.S.

The ascending colon, descending colon, and proximal rectum are covered on the anterior surface and some parts of the lateral surface by peritoneum. The serosa does not protect the posterior surface of the colon. This surface is in direct contact with the retroperitoneal structures. The transverse and sigmoid colons are entirely within the peritoneal cavity covered, circumferentially, by the peritoneum, whereas the distal rectum is totally retroperitoneal.

Injuries to the transverse and sigmoid colons and anterior injuries to the ascending and descending segments of the colon are diagnosed and managed as any other intra-abdominal gastrointestinal (GI) tract injury. The retroperitoneal portions of the colon cannot mount an immediate peritoneal inflammatory response. Therefore injuries to these segments are much more difficult to diagnose. Retroperitoneal injuries that leak do not produce early symptoms, and therefore the abscesses that are formed produce only minimal early signs. These injuries are only diagnosed by the detection of the abscess when early exploration has not been performed. The lack of early signs is characteristic of retroperitoneal GI injuries. The evaluation process must be different for these hidden wounds.

Management of colon trauma during the 1970s and into the early 1980s was unchanged from the end of World War II, in spite of rumblings of new information. All colon penetrations were treated with a colostomy. In the 1990s the colon will be treated the same as the small bowel, although military acceptance of these new principles will be slow and difficult, as demonstrated by the war in the Persian Gulf.

ANATOMY

The colon begins on the right side of the abdomen as the terminal ileum enters the cecum through the ileocecal valve. More often than not, the cecum is a partially retroperitoneal structure from the beginning. As the colon turns across the abdomen at the hepatic flexure, it usually becomes entirely an intra-abdominal organ. At the tip of the spleen, the colon turns caudad and again becomes a structure covered on only part of its surface by peritoneum. The descending colon continues in this fashion until it becomes an intra-abdominal structure for a variable distance (sigmoid colon). Approximately 25 cm from the anus, the colon begins to burrow under the peritoneum. It remains partially within the peritoneal cavity for roughly 10 cm, and then 15 cm from the anus it loses all contact with the peritoneum (Fig. 10–1).

The blood supply to the colon is through a series of arches that are branches of the superior mesenteric artery (Fig. 10–2). The ileocolic artery and several branches, known as right colic arteries, provide blood supply to the right colon and the hepatic flexure. Somewhere along the right colon, these arches will coalesce to form a single marginal artery of Drummond. This vessel runs from that point to the rectum, picking up additional blood from the middle colic artery. It terminates as the superior hemorrhoidal artery and supplies the proximal rectum. Adding supplementary blood supply to the marginal artery along the left colon is the inferior mesenteric artery. This artery is a single branch of the aorta. The middle hemorrhoidal and inferior hemorrhoidal arteries supply the rectum from below and the sides and anastomose to the superior hemorrhoidal artery. This series of vessels protects the colon from ischemia by providing collateral flow, if any of the vessels are blocked. In general, interruption of inferior mesenteric artery in the young trauma patient will not compromise colon blood supply.

ASSESSMENT

One of the more critical components in the management of any injury, and particularly colon injuries with isolated retroperitoneal trauma, is the identification of the injury or assuring that it is not present. Penetrating wounds of the back that do not penetrate the

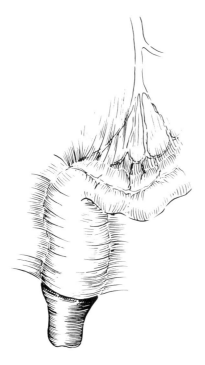

Figure 10–1. The rectum becomes a partial retroperitoneal organ at approximately 25 cm from the anus, but it is covered on its anterior surface by the peritoneum. At 15 cm from the rectum, it is a totally retroperitoneal organ and without serosa.

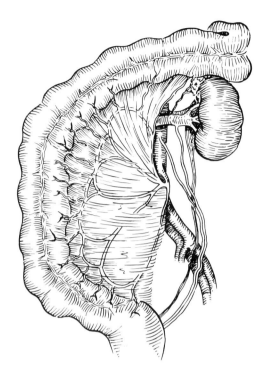

Figure 10–2. The blood supply to the colon is from a series of arch vessels terminating in the single anterior rectal artery as an extension of the marginal artery of Drummond which supplies the superior rectum. Paired medial and inferior rectal arteries provide blood supply from below.

peritoneal cavity but do injure the retroperitoneal organs will neither produce early peritoneal signs nor a positive peritoneal lavage. The computed tomography (CT) scan, although very helpful in identifying solid organ injury, does not prove particularly beneficial in the diagnosis of such injuries, either.

As has been amply taught by the classic work of Cope,[1] there is no pain innervation to the peritoneum. The peritoneum's only sensory response is to stretching. Stretch of the peritoneum, initiated by peritoneal inflammation, is perceived by the brain as pain. In the retroperitoneal portion of the colon there is no peritoneal lining, therefore no early pain response. Injuries to this portion of the colon are not appreciated by the usual signs and symptoms of an acute abdomen. If no other methods of identification are used, the colon perforation is only detected several days later when the abscess has enlarged to reach the peritoneal lining or the inflammation of the muscles in the vicinity becomes significant.

Retroperitoneal leakage becomes an even more difficult assessment problem in the bluntly traumatized abdomen and injuries associated with cervical cord injury. Soderstrom et al[2] reviewed a group of such patients. Of 288 patients with cord injuries, 69% were not in neurogenic shock. Twelve (4.2%) had intra-abdominal injuries, three of which were in shock. Of the patients with intra-abdominal, all injuries were detectable by peritoneal lavage. Of the 58 patients in neurogenic shock, three were found to have associated intra-abdominal injuries but the physical examination of the abdomen in all patients was noncontributory to diagnosis.[2]

Peritoneal Lavage

Peritoneal lavage can be a very effective technique with intra-abdominal injuries. Since the initial description of diagnostic peritoneal lavage (DPL) by Root et al,[3] there has not been a more accurate or a more useful test to determine the presence of organ damage in the patient with blunt trauma. Their report of 97% accuracy (1% false-negative and 2% false-positive results) has held up despite multiple other reviews of its effectiveness. Thal,[4] however, in reviewing 123 patients with lower chest and abdominal penetrating wounds from Parkland Hospital, found that small bowel perforations were present with red blood cell counts as low as 10,000 red cells/mm^3. Merlotti et al[5] found that, using the standard criteria, 100,000 red cells/mm^3, there was a 11.1% false-negative rate. When 50,000 cells/ml^3 were used, the false-negative rate was a unacceptable 9.3%. Only if 10,000 cells/ml^3 were used could diagnostic peritoneal lavage be effective in determining penetrating trauma. The detection rate of retroperitoneal penetrating injuries is even more inaccurate with this test.

Computerized Tomography

The CT scan has been recommended as an effective device for the evaluation of the retroperitoneal space. The general use of this technique for the evaluation of retroperitoneal injury is discussed in Chapter 4. For the retroperitoneal portion of the colon, the use is very limited.

MANAGEMENT

The literature in the last decade is replete with articles discussing the three most often suggested techniques for management of colon injuries: primary suture (including resection and anastomosis), exteriorized repair of the colon wound, and colostomy.

In modern history we give the initiative for primary closure rather than colostomy to Woodhall and Ochsner,[6] who reported on the success of this technique in 1951. A much earlier reference, however, comes from the classic book "Memories of Military Surgeons" by Baron Dominique Jean Larrey, M.D. This book was first translated into English in 1814. In discussing his campaigns in Egypt and Syria that began on the 13th of May, 1798, Dr. Larrey described "the sigmoid curve of the colon was often wounded, and the wounds were cured without leaving an artificial anus. We had two such cases at the siege of Acre and two at Cairo. I took care to dilate the parts where the ball made its entry and its exit."[7]

The fatality rate from gunshot wounds to the intestine and colon throughout military history has been significant. During the War between the States, or the War of Northern Aggression (1861–1865), wounds of the abdomen carried a mortality rate of 90%. During World War I the mortality rate was 60% (Table 10–1). The morality was unchanged in the first part of World War II. Responding to these disastrous results, an edict came from the Surgeon General's office declaring that all wounds of the colon would be initially treated by colostomy.[8] Ogilvie[9] discussed the wisdom of this decision. His personal opinion was that all colon wounds should be treated with a colostomy; however, the data that he reported do not bear out the conclusion, with mortality of suture alone being 44%, and mortality of

Table 10–1   Colon Injury Mortality

STUDY	%
War Between the States (1861–1865)	90.0
Spanish American (1812)	62.5
World War I (1914–1918)	59.6
Charity Hospital (1927–1942)	67.5
Elkin and Ward (1943)	55.5
World War II	31.4
Korean Conflict (1950–1953)	15.0
Grady Hospital (1950–1960)	18.1
Charity Hospital (1943–1958)	13.1
Sanders (1963)	14.0
Louisville General Hospital (1973–1975)	12.9
Grady Hospital (1961–1965)	8.3
Charity Hospital (1959–1974)	9.2
San Francisco General (1970–1975)	3.25
Loma Linda University (1956–1962)	14.5
Bogota, Colombia (1981–1983)	1.9
Lincoln Medical Center (1976–1985)	3.5
Denver General Hospital (1977–1983)	3.0
Detroit Receiving Hospital (1980–1987)	2.5

colostomy and suture being 45%. In 1945 Colcock[10] added more data. Cutler[11] described how such information gained during wartime experience should be translated into civilian medicine. The reduction in mortality to 30% after institution of this practice in the African campaign has been used to vindicate the decision. In 1951 Woodhall and Ochsner[6] first questioned this dogma and suggested that certain injuries could be closed with an improved outcome. Reports by Pontius et al[12] and Roof et al[13] expanded on this concept. In 1963 Vannix et al[14] reported a mortality rate of 6.6% when primary closure was used, 10% when exteriorization was used, and 23.9% when colostomy or cecostomy was used. The mortality was 50% when no surgical treatment at all was performed.[14]

In 1963, 34 patients were reviewed from the Texas Medical Center Hospital, of which 18 patients were treated with primary closure (three deaths), nine patients, with initial anastomosis (no deaths), and five patients, with exteriorizations (one death). Only one of these four deaths (exteriorization) was thought to be related to the colon injury and method of repair. In 1971, 71 right colon injuries were reported from Cook County Hospital.[15] Patients with a primary repair had a total of 41% intra-abdominal abscesses, 33% associated with stab wounds and 50% associated with gunshot wounds. Exteriorized wounds carried an intra-abdominal abscess rate of zero with an average of 14 days in the hospital, whereas the average stay for the primary closure group was 21 days. For a right hemicolectomy after gunshot wounds, there was a 12.5% intra-abdominal abscess rate with 26.7 average days in the hospital, and with a tube cecostomy or colostomy, the intra-abdominal abscess rate was 25% with 15.5 days in the hospital. Haynes et al[16] in 1968 noted a mortality decrease from 18% in the years 1950 through 1960 to 8.3% in 1961 through 1965 at Grady Hospital in Atlanta. The authors thought that primary closure should only be used in small puncture wounds and that all other wounds should be treated by a colostomy either at the injury site or proximal. In 1973, from the Vietnam conflict, 13 patients were reported whose wounds were closed primarily and exteriorized.[17] The colon in 12 of the 13 patients was reduced back into the abdomen at 8 days.

In the largest series up to that time, LoCicero et al[18] in 1975 reported on 50 years' experience with colon injuries at Charity Hospital. The change in philosophy toward more primary repairs and the reduced morbidity rate over these years are seen in Table 10–2. These authors suggested that selected use of primary repair is an important consideration, since lower mortality, fewer complications, and a shorter hospital stay are associated with this technique.

Steele and Blaisdell,[19] in reviewing 5 years' experience (124 patients) from San Francisco General Hospital, found 3.25% of deaths related to bowel injuries. They thought that the data demonstrated that there was no difference in complications, mortality rate, or infection rate when primary repairs of the left colon were compared to similar repairs of the right colon. Colostomy was associated with no deaths and 23% infection rate, primary repair, with 8% deaths and 20% infection rate, and a 15% death rate and 54% infection rate with resection and anastomosis. The authors believed that both the right and left colon should be treated similarly. In reviewing the article, Freeark agreed.[20] In this same issue, Matolo and Wolfman[21] stated that primary repair should be used if peritoneal contamination is minimal. In 1985 a review of the Denver General Hospital experience found 17% sepsis with a 1% mortality rate from primary closure, whereas colostomy carried a septic rate of 48% and 2% mortality.[22] This review showed that with a Penetrating Abdominal Trauma Score (PATI) of 25 or less, less than 25% of the circumference of the colon injured (Flint Score II), and with minimal fecal contamination primary anastomosis had a more favorable outcome. These patients did not do better with a colostomy.

In a nonrandomized but similarly injured series of patients, over 7 years at San Francisco General Hospital, primary closure versus colostomy was compared.[23] They found a mortality rate of 2.6% in each group, but 11% morbidity in the primary closure group and 49% in the colostomy group. When the specific group of PATI was greater than 25, Flint score was 2 or more and Injury Severity Scale was greater than 25, significant complications occurred with the primary closure. These authors believed that PATI was the most reliable predictor of complications and specifically identified patients whose outcome would be better with primary repair. They also identified an increase in complication rate when more than 4 U of blood was required for transfusion and when there was a high degree of fecal spillage. There was no difference in complications between right and transverse versus left and sigmoid colon.

In 1990, a study from Detroit Receiving Hospital reviewed a 7-year experience with colon injuries.[24] Patients with primary closure had a 4.7% incidence of intra-abdominal abscess, whereas patients with colostomy had an abscess rate of 12% (statistically significant difference). Exteriorization of the primary repair resulted in a 33% intra-

Table 10–2   Charity Hospital Management*

	1927–1942	1943–1958	1959–1974
Primary repair	0	39%	44%
Repair and proximal colostomy	0	13%	22%
Colostomy at injury site	100%	48%	33%

*Modified from LoCicero et al.[18]

abdominal abscess rate. The authors thought that preoperative shock and a higher PATI were associated with increased intra-abdominal abscesses.

In 1979 a prospective study demonstrated that shock, hemorrhage, and degree of contamination could be analyzed to identify those patients who would significantly benefit from primary repair rather than colostomy.[25]

Cohn et al[26] randomized 54 patients in a primary closure or primary anastomosis versus colostomy study. Twenty-seven were diverted (24 colostomy, ileostomy, and jejuneostomy) and 27 were closed. There was no difference in the initial results; however, the readmission for closure significantly changed the outcome toward better results for primary closure. There were no leakages from the primary suture line. Volume of transfusion, PATI, and shock influenced the outcome. They concluded that primary closure or primary anastomosis should be the procedure of choice for all colon injuries.

In reviewing the problem from a different prospective, Naraynsingh et al[27] studied 161 consecutive colon injuries in a developing country where colostomy produced a cultural or logistic disadvantage. Of these patients, 93 had a primary closure done, and there was only one anastomotic leakage and 10% infection rate. This is comparable to other studies that have reviewed the infectious results of primary closure.[26–29]

Although there will be some differences of opinions and philosophies, in the early 1990s, at least the most experienced trauma surgeons will agree that at the time of primary operations, there is very little difference in the outcome of primary closure or primary anastomosis versus colostomy. The increased complication rate comes with the additional problems encountered with the closure of the colostomy. This was first pointed out by Moore et al,[28] and expanded on by Ridgeway et al.[29] In the latter study from Charity Hospital at New Orleans, there was an increased complication rate of 33% at the time of closure and added mortality of 2%. The closures were done by upper level house officers, with staff supervision. The overall difference in the two procedures was shown to be: Days in hospital, 10 ± 3 versus 26 ± 4 ($p < 0.05$), and complications, 20% versus 27% (NS).

These two studies and the Cohn et al[26] study reported at the Southern Surgical Association Meeting in 1990 all have similar outcomes, demonstrating that the problem of colostomy adding to the overall outcome of patients with colon injuries is not a localized phenomenon.

Colostomy does increase the complications and the mortality because of the needed second procedure for the colostomy closure. Both factors must be considered when evaluating the outcome of the original operation.

The approach for the management of colon injuries, especially retroperitoneal, should be selective, as it is for injuries in other regions of the body. This protocol is based on the just-described literature and 13 years' experience in a major trauma center (4100 trauma admissions in 1989) whose patient load is 85% penetrating trauma (Fig. 10–3).

Management of penetrating wounds to the colon should be simple closure or resection and primary anastomosis unless one or more of the following conditions are met:

1. High energy, military injuries or shrapnel
2. Abdominal trauma index greater than 25 (multiple other organs injured)
3. More than 4 units of blood administered to the patient
4. Persistent shock prior to or during surgery
5. Prolonged time from injury to operative repair (more than 24 hours)

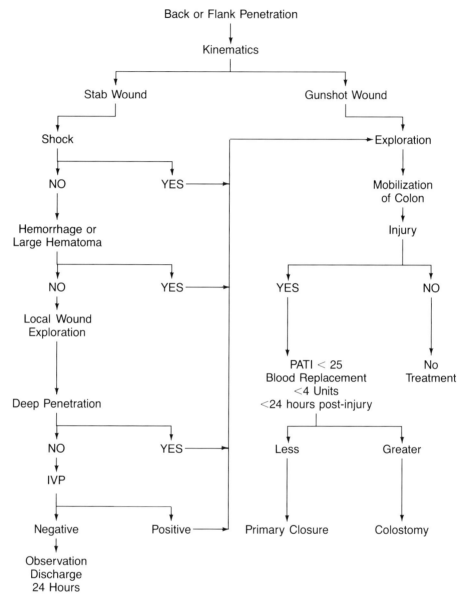

Figure 10–3.   Protocol for colon evaluation and management. IVP: intravenous pyelogram; PATI: Penetrating Abdominal Trauma Index.

When these conditions are exceeded, colostomy should be strongly considered, although not mandated.

There seems to be very little place for exteriorization of a repaired wound. The colostomy itself may be exteriorization of the wound site, but exteriorization of the repair site has not been demonstrated to be effective. The flow chart gives colon trauma decision-making recommendations (Fig. 10–3).

OPERATIVE ASSESSMENT

Mobilization of the right colon to visualize the retroperitoneal surface, is executed by incising the lateral peritoneal reflection (white line of Toldt). The inferior component of the incision begins at the cecum. This incision is carried to the hepatic flexure. Reflecting the colon medially will expose the iliac vessels, the vena cava, the kidney, and on the opposite side, the aorta as well as the important nonserosal covered colon (retroperitoneal colon).

Similarly, on the left side, incising the white line of Toldt and reflecting the colon medially will reveal the left iliac vessels, the aorta, the vena cava (on the right side), the kidneys and renal vessels and the retroperitoneal colon. The inferior mesentery artery will usually be reflected medially with the left colon and can be found in close approximation to the peritoneum between the left colon and the aorta. These two maneuvers allow visual evaluation of the retroperitoneal portion of the colon. No other technique assures that this portion of the colon is uninjured. It should be performed in any patient with an injury in the vicinity.

Another reason for mobilization of the colon is to evaluate, protect, and repair, if necessary, the ureter. Reflection of the ureter is not as consistent, however. This connection between the kidney and the bladder may stay along the retroperitoneal surface in close proximity to the psoas muscle or it may adhere to the underside of the peritoneum and be mobilized medially within the fat of this pseudomesentery. Recognition of which direction the ureter moves is necessary to prevent damage to it.

Exposure of the retroperitoneal rectum is achieved by incising the peritoneum around the lateral and anterior surfaces of the rectum as it reflects from the lateral walls of the abdominal cavity and along the inferior border of the urinary bladder. Blunt dissection with the fingers can be carried out anteriorly and posteriorly, but should not be done on the lateral sides unless absolutely necessary. Damage to the middle or inferior hemorrhoidal vessels should be avoided if possible.

Intraoperative Autotransfusion

With the possibility of blood-borne and blood transmittable diseases such as the acquired immunodeficiency syndrome or hepatitis, and with the relatively poor outcome carried by these conditions, utilization of the patient's own blood for management is important.

Autotransfusion was revived by Grady Hospital in the late 1960s by Symbas.[30] Although autotransfusion had been used many years earlier dating back as far as the early 1900s, there had been minimal use of this approach for almost 50 years. With the successful use of blood scavenger and autotransfusion in cardiothoracic cases, and with the impetus of autotransfusion in thoracic trauma, the use of autotransfusion in intra-abdominal injuries seemed logical. Beginning in 1980 at Charity Hospital in New Orleans, on the Tulane surgical services, we started using autotransfusion for abdominal trauma, whether or not GI tract injuries were present. Initial analysis did not identify a significant increase of major infections or sepsis. One short time frame was reported.[31]

The use of contaminated blood for autotransfusion did not increase the systemic infection rate as identified by generalized sepsis, intrahepatic abscesses, renal infections, or pneumonia when the patients were given preoperative, intraoperative, and postoperative antibiotics. A prospective group of 152 patients with penetrating abdominal trauma and intestinal injury was analyzed, in 20 patients of whom contaminated autotransfused blood and a PATI more than 20 was used and was compared to similar patients with a PATI more than 20 who received banked blood alone.[32]

The use of fecally contaminated but washed autotransfused blood did not increase the incidence of infections, either systemic or local, over patients similarly stratified based on PATI. Although all blood was exposed to the fecal contamination, 85 to 86% of the reinfused blood was culture sterile at the time of reinfusion. The use of such blood scavaged from the traumatized abdomen reduced the need for banked blood by 37%. In this time of decreased blood donations, centrifuged and washed autotransfused blood produces a major resource savings while not introducing an increased infection or complications rate.

The use of such blood has also been examined with attention to coagulation factors. Although most coagulation factors have been washed free, the use of such blood does not increase the loss of clotting factors beyond that expected and found with use of banked blood alone. The coagulation difficulties produced by such massive reinfusions are secondary to washout of the existing factors.[33] Almost all of the blood infused in trauma patients today is packed red blood cells, the clotting factors having been spun off to be given as factor replacement. The only difference in autotransfused blood is that it has been washed also. The outcome with regard to clotting factors is the same. One other consideration is residual heparin, which was used as the anticoagulant. In this same study, ten consecutive patients had heparin levels measured in the blood reinfused and 2 hours postoperatively. No heparin was found.

Antibiotics

Use of antibiotics is critical in the trauma patient. Several studies have emphasized the need for preoperative and intraoperative antibiotics and appropriate postoperative continuation of them.[22,34] A single broad-spectrum antibiotic with good aerobic and anaerobic coverage has been demonstrated to be effective unless a specific culturable bacteria is grown that would indicate necessary change.[34] The length of time that the antibiotic is continued postoperatively depends on the amount of contamination, number of organs injured, amount of blood loss, and length of hypoperfusion. Antibiotics are best continued for 5 days if there are multiple organs injured and significant shock has been present.

Morbidity of Colostomy

Unfortunately, outcome at the time of discharge from the hospital does not give the true picture of the complications and mortality of a colostomy. When creation of the colostomy alone is considered, the data are weighted toward primary closure in selected patients in a small but important way. When the morbidity and mortality of the colostomy closure are added to the equation, the balance shifts much more dramatically toward primary closure. From the University of Texas Health Science Center, a postoperative complication rate of 10% was associated with a colostomy closure reported in 1980.[35] In their article the authors reviewed several other studies from 1975 to 1979 with morbidity rates ranging from 7.4 to 28% at the time of the closure (average of all series, 17%). From Charity Hospital, retrospective analysis of colostomy closure revealed a 28% morbidity rate with an additional 13 days in the hospital.[29] Denver General Hospital reported an additional 24% complications during colostomy closure.[22,28] These data point out the fact that the surgical management must take into consideration the complications of follow-up hospitalizations and procedures in planning the initial treatment. In the specific case of a colostomy, the significant morbidity and mortality of the takedown procedure should make the surgeon think twice before bringing the colon onto the abdominal wall.

Selective Management

Posterior abdominal penetrating trauma represents the unique diagnostic challenge for the reasons already defined. Several studies have addressed this problem. Peck and Berne,[36] treating stab wounds, identified that using chest radiograph, intravenous pyelogram (IVP), and abdominal examination in conjunction with a complete blood count, urinalysis, and serum amylase, 80% of the patients did not require surgery. IVP was done on 34% of the patients for gross or microscopic hematuria, or proximity of injury. Significant organ injury was found in 14%, and 6% had negative laparotomy. Of those patients with significant organ injury, the colon was injured more than any other organ (40%) with the stomach, liver, diaphragm, spleen, and major vessels injured in approximately 20% of the patients. Coppa et al[37] looking at the same problem found a 10% false-negative rate with DPL. With close observation of these patients and with appropriate ancillary studies, such as IVP, selective angiography, and DPL (in spite of the false negatives), selective management was achievable.

Henao et al[38] studied trauma patients in Bogota, Colombia, and thought that all gunshot wounds should be explored, but stab wounds should be managed selectively. Only 30% of the stab wounds were explored based on local exploration, 24 hours of observation, chest and abdominal films, and IVP. The negative exploration rate was kept at 5%. Jackson and Thal[39] found physical examination accurate in 88% of back wounds but not reliable in identifying retroperitoneal injuries.

Grieco and Perry[40] found that of patients with a retroperitoneal hematoma, 65% had significant pathologic conditions that required surgical exploration.

Putting together the available information, assessment of retroperitoneal injuries, and retroperitoneal injuries of the colon in particular, is difficult. Initial physical examination may be unreliable when used alone. There are no diagnostic tests that by itself will provide the definitive answer. Patients who are evaluated in a stepwise manner using the flow chart in Figure 10–3 should allow exploratory laparotomy rate in only 20 to 30% of stab wounds and 100% of gunshot wounds.

The initial evaluation process should address mechanism of injury and shock. If either condition is met, the patient should be immediately taken to the operating room. Local wound exploration should follow. If the wound goes into the posterior abdominal muscles, this should be considered as positive. It is extremely difficult to find out by local exploration the depth of penetration in muscle.

An IVP should be obtained if proximity of the injury or urinalysis increases the suspicion of injury to the ureter, bladder, or kidney.

Rectum

The general philosophy toward no colostomy for colon injuries does not hold for injuries to the rectum. Contamination of the perirectal space, inability to close the injury adequately, and difficulty in diagnosing the extent of injury are all factors that lead to this conclusion.

Diagnosis

Penetrating injuries are diagnosed first by suspicion when the penetrating object was in the general vicinity of where the rectum should be, second by rectal/digital examination, and finally by proctoscopy. In a large report of civilian gunshot wounds, Mangiante et al[41] identified that rectal examinations were positive in 80% of the cases, proctoscopy in 91%, and combined accuracy of 95%. Five percent of injuries cannot be ignored; therefore mandatory abdominal exploration with close attention to the pelvic floor and possible pathway of the missile are important.

Management

The three criteria for managing rectal wounds have been proximal colostomy, presacral drainage, and distal washout.

The type of colostomy does not seem to matter. Loop colostomy or end colostomy with mucous fistula both seem to be acceptable with very similar complication rates. In the previously identified study from Memphis, whether or not presacral drains were used did not seem to affect the outcome; however, lack of use of rectal washout was significant. Of the small number that did not receive the rectal washout, all developed complications, whereas no major intra-abdominal complications occurred in the larger group with rectal washout accomplished.

Lavenson and Cohen[42] also identified that there was a significant reduction in complications with the use of distal washout. In penetrating trauma therefore proximal colostomy and distal rectal washout are extremely important. Presacral drains and the type of colostomy do not seem to matter.

Distal or rectal washout is accomplished by dilating the rectum to allow 3 or 4 fingers to pass with ease. A catheter is then inserted into the distal end of the colostomy and irrigated with normal saline until no fecal material is present and the liquid coming out of the rectum is clear. This is best accomplished after the abdomen has been closed.

If it is possible to close the mucosa on the rectal wound, this most probably should be accomplished. Frequently, the injury can be visualized either through the rectum or by taking down the peritoneum as the rectum proceeds from the abdomen to retroperitoneal space. This repair is done from above in the standard two-layer manner and from below by simply closing the mucosa with continuous sutures. If a significant pelvic hematoma is present, it is best left undisturbed to avoid uncontrollable hemorrhage. Colostomy and distal washout are still performed.

Blunt Trauma

The rectum injured with blunt trauma is usually associated with a fractured pelvis. Diverting colostomy is extremely important in this situation, along with distal washout and closure of the injury to minimize pelvic contamination and infection of the pelvic fracture sites. Again, significant pelvic hematomas are not entered, so loss of tamponade is avoided.

SUMMARY

The majority of the colon is intra-abdominal, but the posterior surface of the ascending and descending colon and most of the rectum are retroperitoneal. Diagnosis is based on a high degree of suspicion and proximity of injury. If doubt exists as to the presence of an injury, exploration is mandated with mobilization of the colon to visualize the posterior surfaces. This is particularly true in penetrating trauma to the back and flank. There are no preoperative diagnostic tests that are reliable. In the majority of civilian trauma patients, primary repair of colon injuries is appropriate. Rectal injuries are managed with diverting colostomy and distal segment washout. Presacral drainage appears to be optional as long as the first two procedures are performed.

REFERENCES

1. Cope Z: *Cope's Early Diagnosis of the Acute Abdomen*, 17th ed. Revised by William Silen. New York: Oxford University Press, 1987.
2. Soderstrom CA, McArdle DQ, Ducker TB, Militello PR: The diagnosis of intra-abdominal injury in patients with cervical cord trauma. *J Trauma* 1983;23:1061–1065.
3. Root HD, Hauser CW, McKinley CR, et al: Diagnostic peritoneal lavage. *Surgery* 1965;57:633–637.
4. Thal ER: Evaluation of peritoneal lavage and local exploration in lower chest and abdominal stab wounds. *J Trauma* 1977;17:642–648.
5. Merlotti GJ, Marcet E, Sheaff CM, Dunn R, Barrett JA: Use of peritoneal lavage to evaluate abdominal penetration. *J Trauma* 1985;25:228–231.
6. Woodhall JP, Ochsner A: The management of perforating injuries of the colon and rectum in civilian practice. *Surgery* 1951;29:305–320.
7. Larrey DJ: *Memories of Military Surgeons and Campaigns of the French Army*. Baltimore, MD: Joseph Cushing, 1914. Republished Birmingham, AL: Graphon Editions, 1985, pp 320–321.
8. Office of the Surgeon General: Circular letter #178, October 23, 1943.
9. Ogilvie WH: Abdominal wounds in the western desert. *Surg Gynecol Obstet* 1944;78:225–238.
10. Colcock BP: Traumatic perforation of the colon as seen in a general hospital. *Surgery* 1945;17:1–10.
11. Cutler CW. Profits to peace-time practice from surgical experiences of war. *Ann Surg* 1945;122:734–743.
12. Pontius RC, Creech O Jr, DeBakey ME: Management of large bowel injuries in civilian practice. *Ann Surg* 1957;146:291–295.
13. Roof WR, Morris GC, DeBakey ME: Management of perforating injuries to the colon in civilian practice. *Am J Surg* 1960;99:641–645.
14. Vannix RS, Carter R, Hinshaw DB, Joergenson EJ: Surgical management of colon trauma in civilian practice. *Am J Surg* 1963;106:364–371.
15. Chilimindris C, Boyd DR, Carlson LE, et al: A critical review of management of right colon injuries. *J Trauma* 1971;11(8).
16. Haynes CD, Gunn CH, Martin JD Jr: Colon injuries. *Arch Surg* 1968;96:944–948.
17. Middleton CJ, Wayne MA: Exteriorization of repaired missile wounds of the colon. *J Trauma* 1973;13: 460–462.
18. LoCicero J III, Tajima T, Drapanas T: A half-century of experience in the management of colon injuries: Changing concepts. *J Trauma* 1975;15:575–587.
19. Steele M, Blaisdell FW: Treatment of colon injuries. *J Trauma* 1977;17:557–562.
20. Freeark RJ: The injured colon (Editorial). *J Trauma* 1977;17:563–564.
21. Matolo NM, Wolfman EF Jr: Primary repair of colonic injuries: A clinical evaluation. *J Trauma* 1977;17:554–556.

22. Shannon FL, Moore EE: Primary repair of the colon: When is it a safe alternative? *Surgery* 1985;98: 851–859.
23. Nelken N, Lewis F: The influence of injury severity on complication rates after primary closure or colostomy for penetrating colon trauma. *Ann Surg* 1989;209:439–447.
24. Levison MA, Thomas DD, Wiencek RG, Wilson RF: Management of the injured colon: Evolving practice at an urban trauma center. *J Trauma* 1990;30:247–253.
25. Stone HH, Fabian TC: Management of perforating colon trauma. Randomization between primary closure and exteriorization. *Ann Surg* 1979;190:430–436.
26. Cohn I, Chappuis CW, Dietzen CD, Frey DJ, Panetta T, Buechter KJ: Management of penetrating colon injuries: A prospective randomized trial. *South Surg Assoc* 1990; 25.
27. Naraynsingh V, Ariyanayagam D, Pooran S: Primary repair of colon injuries in a developing country. *Br J Surg* 1991;78:319–320.
28. Moore EE, Dunn EL, Moore JB, Thompson JS: Penetrating Abdominal Trauma Index. *J Trauma* 1981;21:439–445.
29. Ridgeway CA, Frame SB, Rice JC, Timberlake GA, McSwain NE Jr, Kerstein MD: Primary repair versus colostomy for the treatment of penetrating colon injuries. *Dis Colon Rectum* 1989;32:1046–1049.
30. Symbas PN: Autotransfusion from hemothorax: Experimental and clinical studies. *J Trauma* 1972;12:689.
31. Timberlake GA, McSwain NE Jr: Autotransfusion of blood contaminated by enteric contents: A potentially life-saving measure in the massively hemorrhaging trauma patient. *J Trauma* 1988;28:855–857.
32. McSwain NE Jr, Ozmen V, Nichols RL, Smith J, Flint LM: Autotransfusion of culture-positive blood (CPB) in abdominal trauma. Presented at the Southern Surgical Association meeting, Boca Raton, Florida, December, 1990.
33. McSwain NE Jr, Ozmen V, Englehardt TC, Nichols RL, Smith J, Flint LM: Coagulopathy and autotransfusion, a clinical problem. Presented at Eastern Association for Trauma, Bermuda, January 1992.
34. Nichols RL, Smith JW, Klein DB, et al: Risk of infection after penetrating abdominal trauma. *N Engl J Med* 1984;311:1065–1070.
35. Thal ER, Yeary EC: Morbidity of colostomy closure following colon trauma. *J Trauma* 1980;20:287–291.
36. Peck JJ, Berne TV: Posterior abdominal stab wounds. *J Trauma* 1981;21:298–306.
37. Coppa GF, Davalle M, Pachter NL, Hofsetter SR: Management of penetrating wounds of the back and flank. *Surg Gynecol Obstet* 1984;159:514–518.
38. Henao F, Jimenez H, Tawil M: Penetrating wounds of the back and flank: Analysis of 77 cases. *South Med J* 1987;80:21–25.
39. Jackson GL, Thal ER: Management of stab wounds of the back. *J Trauma* 1979;19:660–664.
40. Grieco JG, Perry JF Jr: Retroperitoneal hematoma following trauma: Its clinical importance. *J Trauma* 1980;20:733–736.
41. Mangiante EC, Graham AD, Fabian TC: Rectal gunshot wounds: Management of civilian injuries. *Am Surg* 1986;52:37–40.
42. Lavenson GS, Cohen A: Management of rectal injuries. *Am J Surg* 1971;122:226–230.

11

Vascular Injuries

R. MARK SAROYAN, M.D.
MORRIS D. KERSTEIN, M.D., F.A.C.S.

Injuries to the vascular system, by blunt or penetrating mechanisms, are the most common serious trauma sustained in the retroperitoneum.[1] By definition, retroperitoneal vascular injuries include injury to the aorta and its major branches, vena cava and its major tributaries, portal and hepatic veins, and pelvic vasculature.

The majority of major retroperitoneal vascular injuries presenting to busy inner city trauma centers are penetrating and carry a high mortality rate, ranging from 35 to 49%.[2-4] This high rate of hospital mortality reflects the magnitude of the injury, frequency of serious associated injuries,[2] and improved prehospital emergency care,[4] allowing successful transport of many injuries that were previously fatal at the scene. Irreversible shock with failure to control hemorrhage is the primary cause of early mortality in both blunt and penetrating injuries of this nature.

At centers dealing with primarily blunt trauma, pelvic fracture is the most common cause of retroperitoneal hematoma,[5] followed by renal injuries. Mortality rates for severe pelvic fractures can reach 50%.[6,7] The chief cause of early mortality is exsanguination. Disability is a reflection of severe associated neurologic injury; therefore the primary concern in initial management of a major pelvic fracture is control of hemorrhage.

DIAGNOSIS AND INITIAL RESUSCITATION

These topics are presented together because most often they must occur simultaneously. Patients arriving in shock (systolic blood pressure less than 90 mmHg) do not allow for an extensive evaluation. Hemodynamic instability can be the result of any one or more concurrent injuries, including retroperitoneal or abdominal vascular trauma, pelvic fracture, long bone fracture, chest trauma, and (as a diagnosis of exclusion) neurologic injury. In the patient with evidence of blood loss, the possibility of significant abdominal or retroperitoneal hemorrhage must be assessed rapidly, and associated injuries confirmed or ruled out. Physical examination and chest radiograph with placement of tube thoracostomy as required can rapidly exclude the thorax as a source of continuing blood loss. The possibility of pericardial tamponade may be assessed quickly by pericardiocentesis or measurement of central venous pressure, if clinically suspected. Long bone and pelvic fractures can be evaluated rapidly by appropriate plain films.

In patients who are extremely unstable, the only hope for salvage may lie in immediate celiotomy for control of hemorrhage from intra-abdominal injuries, despite the knowledge that most of the blood loss may well be retroperitoneal from the pelvic fracture. Results from operative attempts at control of this form of hemorrhage have been, for the most part, dismal.[6,8–10] Patients with severe hypotension (less than 60 mmHg) refractory to maximal efforts at volume resuscitation may require thoracotomy for control of the descending aorta, either in the emergency department (ED) or on arrival to the operating room.[3,11] The specific indications for, and appropriate timing of this maneuver remain highly controversial.[2,4,12,13] There is general agreement, however, that when thoracotomy is required in the ED for this indication (blunt abdominal or pelvic trauma), survival is exceedingly poor (0% to 3%).[3,12] When possible, this maneuver is best reserved for the operating room where celiotomy for definitive control of hemorrhage can proceed immediately after clamping the aorta.

The most frequently difficult therapeutic dilemma occurs in the marginally stable patient who has sustained a concurrent pelvic fracture and possible abdominal injuries. These are patients who respond to aggressive fluid therapy, but continue to require ongoing resuscitation to maintain their blood pressure. An unnecessary celiotomy in this situation delays more definitive therapy and can exacerbate bleeding by release of an extraperitoneal tamponade. An extremely useful test in this setting is open diagnostic peritoneal lavage.[6,14] Positive lavage results must be interpreted with caution; the increased incidence of false-positive lavage in the presence of pelvic fracture is well-documented and is reported at approximately 25 to 29%.[14–16] This has been attributed to diapedesis of red blood cells across the peritoneal membrane from the pelvic hematoma, as well as violation of the hematoma by the lavage catheter as it dissects up the lower abdominal wall. False-positive results can be minimized by careful use of the open supraumbilical technique.[17,18] Gross blood returning on initial aspiration of the lavage catheter or bloody lavage fluid (greater than 100,000 red blood cells/ml) on return remains an indication for immediate celiotomy. Return of clear or only slightly tinged lavage fluid indicates life-threatening intra-abdominal blood loss is unlikely to be the source of continued hypotension, and efforts should be directed toward other means of controlling hemorrhage from the pelvic injury.[6] These maneuvers will be discussed later in Chapter 13.

MANAGEMENT OF SPECIFIC INJURIES

Injuries of the Inferior Vena Cava and Hepatic Veins

Despite advances in prehospital care and surgical techniques of exposure and vascular isolation, injuries to the vena cava continue to generate formidable mortality figures, ranging from 30 to 53% overall in recent literature.[19–22] Mortality rates vary considerably, depending on location of the injury, associated injuries, mechanism of injury (blunt or penetrating), and condition of the patient on arrival at the ED.[19,21–23]

Management of injuries to the vena cava differs considerably, depending on location. For purposes of discussion, injuries to the inferior vena cava can be divided into four segments, based on relationship to the renal veins and liver: infrarenal, pararenal, suprarenal, and retrohepatic.

Despite their surgical accessibility, mortality rates from injuries to the infrarenal vena cava, almost uniformly secondary to penetrating trauma, are surprisingly high, at 17 to 51% in recent series.[20–23] This mortality has been attributed primarily to the condition of the patient on arrival at the hospital and associated major vascular injuries, because surgical exposure at this level is not extremely difficult.

Exposure of the infrarenal vena cava is most conveniently obtained by dividing the lateral peritoneal reflection along the right paracolic gutter and reflecting the right colon medially, which provides good exposure from below the renal veins to the bifurcation. Alternatively, this area can be approached medially, dividing the root of the small bowel mesentery, incising from the ileocecal area to the ligament to Trietz to expose the vena cava.[23] This approach is more cumbersome and used less commonly.

Initial control of the injury is obtained by gentle pressure with a stick sponge, which avoids further trauma to the vessel. Often simple pressure with stick sponges proximal and distal to an anterior or lateral injury allows adequate hemostasis to complete a lateral repair. If this is not successful, the vessel may be gently mobilized proximally and distally, and occluded with vascular clamps, Rumel tourniquets, or a partial occluding Satinsky clamp may be applied at the site of the injury. Care should be taken to avoid further injury to the vessel during this maneuver. Hypotension with caval occlusion at this level indicates the need for further volume resuscitation, and may be treated temporarily by infrarenal aortic occlusion while caval repair is carried out.[3] A careful examination for the presence of a posterior injury should be performed. Frequently, this may be accomplished by examining the lumen before anterior repair. If further doubt exists, the vessel may be mobilized carefully after repair of the anterior injury. Often, this will require the division of one or more lumbar veins. In patients who are hemodynamically stable, large defects in the vessel may be repaired with a patch technique using either saphenous vein or prosthetic material, depending on the degree of contamination and size of the defect. Patients who are unstable, have a severe coagulopathy, and other major vascular injuries in need of control are better served by caval ligation, rather than an extended vascular reconstruction of a complex injury.[22–24] Long-term complications of this maneuver may include lower extremity edema, postphlebitic syndrome, or pulmonary emboli.

Management of injuries to the vena cava at the level of the renal veins is more complex and carries a higher mortality, because of the decreased ability to mobilize the cava in this location, and frequent concomitant injury to one or both of the renal veins. Exposure of this injury is obtained via a generous Kocher maneuver, reflecting the duodenum and head of the pancreas medially. If injury to the cava at the level of the renal veins is strongly suspected, it may be advisable to obtain control of the left renal vein from the midline, anterior to the aorta, and exposure of the infrarenal cava below, by reflecting the hepatic flexure, before the Kocher maneuver.

As the injury is exposed, hemorrhage will occur which may be managed initially by pressure with a stick sponge. Each renal vein is then carefully identified and encircled with vascular loops for control. Mobilization of the cava in this location is difficult, and control above and below the injury is most safely obtained with pressure using stick sponges, because of the presence of the renal veins (Fig. 11–1). If this is unsatisfactory, further mobilization is required for control above and below with vascular clamps or tourniquets. Partial occluding clamps are usually not useful because this will frequently cause, or worsen, a tear to the renal veins.

Lateral venorrhaphy is the technique used most commonly for repair. This often results in mild-to-moderate narrowing of the cava (less than 50%), which is acceptable. If lateral

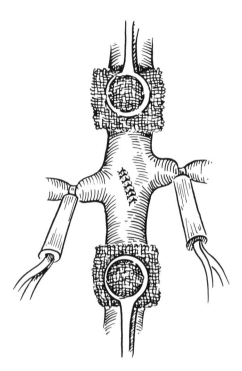

Figure 11–1.   Technique for vascular control of pararenal vena cava injury.

repair results in severe stenosis, a patch technique is recommended, if the patient's condition allows. A concomitant posterior injury to the cava may be considerably more difficult to expose and repair in this location. The possibility of a posterior injury may often be assessed intraluminally, as already described. Repair can be performed intraluminally as well, by extending the anterior injury enough for adequate exposure.[22,23] In the absence of active bleeding or an expanding hematoma, several authors recommend no further mobilization or attempts at repair of a posterior injury that cannot be done easily from an anterior approach.[19,20,23] In a recent series by Stewart and Stone,[20] five patients with posterior nonbleeding caval injuries in whom circumferential dissection of the cava was avoided were successfully managed in this fashion.

Concomitant renal vein injuries should be repaired when possible, either by lateral venorrhaphy or patch technique, as the situation dictates. As with the vena cava, ligation remains an option of last resort. The left renal vein may be ligated with an excellent chance of normal renal function, because of collateral drainage via the left adrenal and gonadal veins.[25] Ligation of the right renal vein has an increased chance of yielding renal dysfunction or hypertension, because it lacks these natural collaterals.

Small lacerations, less than 1 cm, to the suprarenal vena cava below the liver may be controlled initially by finger pressure after exposure via Kocher maneuver. Repair may then be accomplished using a vascular suture with a needle of appropriate size, passing beneath the finger, occluding the defect, and coapting both edges. Partial occluding clamps may be of use, but great care must be taken to avoid further injury in this location. The use of this maneuver is limited because of the proximity of the liver and renal veins. Complete occlusion of the vena cava above and below the injury is also difficult for the same reason and is, in general, poorly tolerated by an already traumatized, hypovolemic patient. Ligation of the vena cava at this level is reserved only as a desperate measure, because survival is infrequent.[23,24] Larger, more complex lacerations extending up to or behind the liver, therefore, may require vascular isolation of the liver, as will be described for retro-hepatic injuries.

Retrohepatic vena caval injuries and hepatic vein injuries are among the most difficult to manage. Attempts at exposure of the injury even for initial assessment are often met with torrential hemorrhage. Associated severe liver and vascular injuries frequently serve to compound the problem. Thus, reported mortality rates for these injuries range from 52 to 100% for blunt injuries and 66 to 87% for penetrating trauma.[3,20,21] The wide variety of surgical approaches for these lesions seen in the literature, most of which report similar mortality figures, attests to the fact that no single method of management is ideal. Treatment should be individualized, depending on both the particular injury and surgeon's familiarity with the various operative approaches.

Major injury to the retrohepatic vena cava or hepatic veins may be suspected by brisk venous bleeding from behind the liver, from a deep parenchymal injury, or a large retrohepatic hematoma, which might also extend onto the diaphragm or inferiorly behind the duodenum. Initial management should include temporizing measures to reduce the bleeding and allow adequate volume resuscitation before attempts at obtaining better exposure. This may include placing laparotomy packs behind the liver and compressing the liver to tamponade the bleeding. Occlusion of the porta hepatis with a vascular clamp, the Pringle maneuver, should be performed, and will be effective at this stage if the bleeding is primarily arterial (that is, from a deep parenchymal injury). A successful Pringle maneuver precludes the need for further hepatic vascular isolation.

If a significant retrohepatic injury is suspected, improved exposure is essential for assessment and repair. Excellent exposure is obtained by extending the celiotomy incision into the chest, either as a median sternotomy or right thoracoabdominal incision. The sternotomy provides easier access to the right atrium if intraluminal shunting is planned and is usually better tolerated by the patient postoperatively.[21,23,26] The diaphragm may then be divided either centrally through the mainly tendinous portion, or circumferentially; both incisions spare the phrenic innervation. Care must be taken as the incision nears the vena cava because the tendinous diaphragm in this area abruptly gives way to the vena cava.[21] The right and left lobes of the liver are then mobilized under direct vision until the hepatic veins are seen, avoiding further damage to these structures.

Small injuries may then be controlled with direct digital pressure and repaired primarily, accepting a moderate blood loss.[3] Larger or more complex injuries will likely require some form of hepatic vascular isolation to obtain a dry field and perform an adequate repair. Intraluminal shunting may be considered with brisk bleeding refractory to a Pringle maneuver and the following operative findings:

1. Vigorous venous bleeding from within the lesser sac (with an intact portal vein)
2. Bleeding from the posterior aspect of the right lobe
3. A deep parenchymal laceration
4. Hematoma at the diaphragm anteriorly
5. Bleeding from beneath the porta hepatis at the inferior edge of the liver[21]

A variety of different approaches to hepatic isolation have been described in the literature. The most widely used is an intraluminal atriocaval shunt described originally by Schrock et al[27] in 1968. A 36 F chest tube is prepared for use as a shunt by cutting an additional hole approximately 20 cm from the most proximal existing hole, and a clamp is applied to the proximal end of the tube. Above the liver, control of the vena cava is obtained within the pericardium using a Rumel tourniquet. Control is obtained below the liver and above the renal veins in a similar manner. The right atrial appendage is then held in a Satinsky clamp while a 2-0 silk purse string suture is applied. The tip of the appendage is excised, allowing insertion of the distal end of the chest tube to be inserted through the atrium and into the inferior vena cava. The surgeon's hand is placed behind the liver to guide the end of the tube and avoid further laceration of the vena cava or hepatic veins. The tube should be advanced until the newly created hole lies within the atrium. At this point, the original holes will be below the renal veins. The atrial purse string and Rumel tourniquets are then tightened, and a check is made to ensure the previously placed vascular clamp remains on the porta hepatis. This maneuver should obtain adequate vascular isolation of the liver. Some bleeding may persist because of venous tributaries from the right adrenal and inferior phrenic veins, but this should be a fraction of that originally encountered. Common pitfalls of this procedure, which may result in continued heavy blood loss, include:

1. Laceration of the vena cava while obtaining proximal or distal control. This most frequently occurs inferiorly, above the renal veins
2. Exacerbation of the existing injury from failure to guide the tip of the chest tube
3. Misplacement of the proximal (outflow) hole in the chest tube
4. Failure to advance the tube far enough, so that one of the distal holes lies between the tourniquets
5. Late placement of the shunt, resulting in an unsalvageable situation

It cannot be overemphasized that if an intraluminal shunt is contemplated it should be placed early, before development of severe coagulopathy and hypothermia from prolonged hemorrhage; this is the most commonly mentioned error in most retrospective reviews of this procedure.[13,20,21]

Several variations on intraluminal shunting have been used, with varying degrees of success. Use of an endotracheal tube was first described and demonstrated by Yellin et al in 1971[28] and used successfully by Rovito[29] in a recent series of severe blunt hepatic vascular injuries. Another method of shunting, also described by Yellin et al[28] involves placement of an intraluminal shunt via the infrarenal vena cava, after gaining control of the vena cava above and below the liver, as already described. This approach has not gained popularity, because other authors have found the maneuver technically difficult and have been unable to duplicate the original favorable results.[21]

Complete caval occlusion for vascular isolation of the liver has been used by some for controlling hemorrhage in trauma; however, the primary application has been in elective hepatic resections.[30] Despite clamping of the thoracic or subdiaphragmatic aorta, most trauma patients will not tolerate total caval occlusion above the renal veins.[3,23,28]

Intraluminal shunts using balloon catheters, which are inserted via cutdown at the saphenofemoral junction, have also been described.[31] As of this time, these devices have seen only limited clinical use.

Pachter et al,[32] in a recent series, reported successful management of major retro-hepatic venous injuries in five consecutive patients using an operative approach that avoided total caval occlusion or intraluminal shunting. This involved initial control of bleeding via compression of the liver and a Pringle maneuver followed by direct "finger fracture" hepatotomy along the tract of the injury to gain exposure. The vena caval injury was then controlled with a partial occluding clamp, followed by lateral venorrhaphy. Most hepatic vein injuries were ligated in this series, without serious sequelae. The final role of the technique in treatment of this injury awaits further clinical evaluation.

Another method of hepatic isolation that avoids intraluminal shunting or total occlusion has also been used. This involves placement from above and below the liver of partial occluding curved aortic clamps on the retrohepatic vena cava (Fig. 11–2). The maneuver requires division of the diaphragm as described previously, and takedown of both triangular ligaments until the hepatic veins are visualized. The liver is then gently retracted anteriorly and clamps applied. This technique is ideally suited to anterior caval and hepatic vein injuries, particularly of the avulsion type found in blunt trauma.

Injuries to the hepatic veins are repaired, when possible, by lateral venorrhaphy. Generally, the condition of the patient sustaining this injury and short length of the vessel precludes more complex repairs. Lacerations that cannot be handled by lateral repair may be ligated safely, provided the remaining major veins are patent.[26,33]

Patients who have developed significant coagulopathy, hypothermia, or both early in their operative course (particularly with extensive concomitant parenchymal liver injury) may not be candidates for repeated attempts at exposure and definitive repair of a retrohepatic venous injury. If packing with direct pressure is successful in controlling

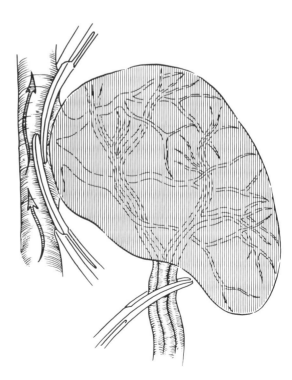

Figure 11–2. Partial occluding clamps on vena cava in association with Pringle maneuver for control of retrohepatic venous injury.

hemorrhage, these patients may be better served by leaving hemostatic packs in place with planned reexploration in 24 to 72 hours. This allows for replacement of coagulation factors and complete rewarming of the patient before removal of the packs. Frequently, at the time of reexploration, no other repair is required other than pack removal. Possible complications of this technique include continued hemorrhage (especially at the time of removing the packs from what may be a large area of denuded liver parenchyma), sepsis, and the morbidity of a second general anesthetic in an already critically ill patient. Clot disruption and further bleeding at the time of pack removal may be minimized by leaving a sterile plastic sheet between the packs and liver at the time of their initial placement. The packs should also be soaked with saline before their gentle removal at the second exploration.

Injuries to the Aorta

The overwhelming majority of injuries to the abdominal aorta are penetrating in nature, most commonly gunshot wounds.[1,3,34] Mortality is considerable, ranging between 50 and 70% in most series.[34–37] This is influenced significantly by the presence of retroperitoneal tamponade (which may prevent exsanguination into the abdominal cavity), by the location of the injury, and other associated vascular injuries.[35,38,39] Millikan and Moore[36] reported a 91% survival in 11 patients with penetrating abdominal aortic injury and an intact retroperitoneal hematoma. The most common associated major vascular injury is to the vena cava, with which survivorship is reported between 0 and 27%.[39,40] In a large collected review, 23% of penetrating aortic injuries had concomitant injuries to the vena cava. Injuries to the suprarenal aorta, in general, carry a higher mortality than those below the renal arteries, because of the more complex surgical exposure and associated injuries to major visceral vessels. Injuries at the level of the diaphragm may be an exception, in that the surrounding diaphragm, as well as dense periaortic neural and lymphatic tissue, encourage a tamponade of the injury.[35]

Injuries of the abdominal aorta may be divided into two main categories, infra- and suprarenal, for purposes of describing operative exposure. Proximal control of the aorta for a suspected suprarenal injury may be obtained immediately below the diaphragm as described previously, or via preliminary left anterolateral thoracotomy for cross-clamping within the left chest, depending on the proximity of the hematoma to the diaphragm. Other available maneuvers include division of the left crus of the diaphragm from within the abdominal cavity, which may provide exposure as high as the ninth thoracic vertebra.[38] The celiotomy may also be extended as a thoracoabdominal incision, with division of the diaphragm circumferentially.

An alternative (although not widely used) method of obtaining proximal aortic control involves passage of a balloon occlusion catheter either from a femoral or brachial approach.

After first obtaining proximal control, the preferred method of exposure involves dividing the left lateral peritoneal reflection, with mobilization of the stomach, spleen, colon, and pancreas toward the midline.[36,38,41] Mattox and associates[41] additionally recommend mobilization of the left kidney, maintaining the plane of dissection on top of the psoas muscle. This results in excellent exposure of the abdominal aorta (and associated visceral vessels) from the ninth thoracic vertebra to the bifurcation. The field of dissection in this plane may be found to be remarkably free of blood, despite a large hematoma more anteriorly. Occasionally, division of the left renal vein may be required for optimal exposure,[35] depending on the location of the injury. Complications of this technique are infrequent, but most commonly include injury to the spleen, pancreas, or lumbar vessels.

Alternate methods of exposure include approach to the injury from below the transverse mesocolon or through the lesser sac. The latter approach involves entrance to the lesser sac through the gastrocolic ligament, with division of the neck of the pancreas to expose the aorta (Fig. 11–3). This may frequently require dissection through a large anterior hematoma. Adequate exposure and control of the injury via either of these approaches is generally more difficult and associated with a higher operative mortality.[38,40]

The majority of penetrating injuries to the suprarenal aorta may be handled by lateral repair.[1,36,39] Generally, only minimal debridement is required before repair with a 3-0 polypropylene vascular suture.[36] Occasionally, large defects may require a patch technique; material for a patch repair may include saphenous vein, hypogastric artery, or polytetrafluorethylene (PTFE) depending on availability, size of the defect, and degree of contamination. In general, autologous material is preferred; however, Feliciano et al[3,39] reported from a large experience that the risk of infection from the use of synthetic conduit is small, even in the presence of gastrointestinal contamination. This topic remains controversial. Complex injuries may require either resection with primary anastomosis or replacement with interposition of a segmental Dacron tube graft, and replantation of major branches as required. Successful revascularization of the renal arteries and superior mesenteric artery has been reported in this setting.[38,40]

Injuries to the celiac axis and proximal superior mesenteric artery are exposed in the same manner as for the suprarenal aorta. Simple lacerations to either of these vessels may be repaired primarily with fine vascular sutures. Complex injuries of the celiac axis or superior mesenteric artery proximal to the edge of the pancreas may be safely ligated in the young trauma patient, because of the extensive collateral circulation.[3] An injury to the superior mesenteric artery distal to the pancreas requires repair or bypass to avoid midgut ischemia.[3]

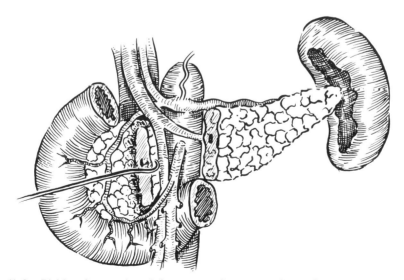

Figure 11–3. Division of pancreatic neck for exposure of retropancreatic vascular structures.

Patch technique may be used for repair, or bypass can be performed from the infrarenal aorta using saphenous vein graft. Bypass from the infrarenal aorta may allow for the reconstruction to be performed in an operative field free from the hematoma of the original injury.

The approach to suspected injuries to the infrarenal aorta is straightforward. Mortality from these injuries is more often from failure of tamponade to develop, resulting in continued hemorrhage, rather than technical problems with exposure. Proximal control initially is obtained immediately below the renal arteries (as for aneurysm repair) or at the diaphragmatic hiatus, depending on the level of the injury. Control may also be obtained via a retroperitoneal approach (as in exposure of a suprarenal injury), cross-clamping the aorta immediately above or below the renal vessels, as required. Distal control is obtained at the proximal common iliac vessels or immediately above the bifurcation. After appropriate exposure and dissection, many lacerations may be isolated with a partial occluding clamp for the repair, allowing restoration of flow distally.

A through-and-through injury to the distal aorta at the bifurcation (which may be accompanied by venous injury to the distal vena cava/iliac confluence) may present a difficult problem in gaining adequate exposure and hemostasis. An occasionally useful technique in this situation involves division of the right common iliac artery, which allows reflection of the distal aorta to the left (Fig. 11–4). Although seldom required, this maneuver may provide excellent exposure of the posterior distal aorta, distal vena cava, and iliac veins.[42]

As in suprarenal injuries, the most common method of management is direct lateral repair. Careful inspection should be made to rule out an occult injury of the opposing aortic wall, either by rotating the vessel after repair of the anterior injury or inspection from within

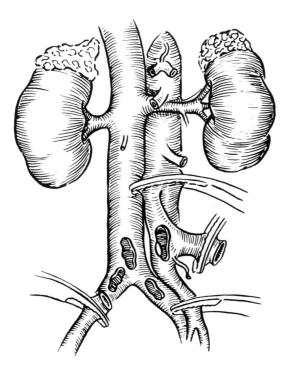

Figure 11–4. Complex aortic and vena caval injuries with right iliac artery divided to improve exposure.

before the repair. Patch technique, resection and primary anastomosis, or prosthetic interposition grafting may be performed for complex injuries as required. As alluded to earlier, appropriate management in the presence of concomitant gastrointestinal injuries is controversial. In the presence of gross contamination, Brinton et al[35] recommend extra-anatomic bypass for injuries that would otherwise require repair with a prosthesis.

Blunt trauma resulting in injury to the abdominal aorta is unusual.[43,44] A recent review of the English literature disclosed only 33 cases diagnosed in living patients.[44] Combining the studies of Parmley et al[45] and Strassman,[46] only 16 of 347 (5%) blunt aortic injuries involved the abdominal aorta; injuries to the thoracic aorta were 20 times more common.[45,46] Overall mortality is reported at 28%; associated injuries were not found to be a contributing factor, although 55% did have concomitant intra-abdominal injuries.[43,44]

The majority of blunt abdominal injuries are the result of motor vehicle accidents, most commonly related to steering wheel trauma. Compression of the aorta against the spine by a direct mechanical force is believed to be the primary mechanism of injury. In contrast, thoracic aortic injuries are caused by sudden deceleration. The chest wall affords some protection to the suprarenal aorta, because 95% of the reported injuries have been located at or below the renal vessels.[44] Atherosclerosis is also believed by some to be a predisposing factor in the genesis of these injuries.[43] Aortic injuries that may result from direct mechanical force include contusion, intimal disruption, pseudoaneurysm, or true rupture.

Approximately two thirds of these injuries are diagnosed within 24 hours of presentation. In the acute setting, the diagnosis may most frequently be suspected by the onset of ischemic symptoms in the lower extremities. Presentation of a chronic injury may include claudication, chronic abdominal pain, pulsatile mass, or decreased pulses. As in thoracic injuries, the definitive diagnosis is best made by aortography, if the patient's condition allows. Often, the diagnosis is not suspected until the time of celiotomy. If exploration for other indications discloses an aortic contusion or nonexpanding hematoma, urgent post-operative aortography is indicated to confirm the diagnosis and guide definitive repair.[43,44] Delays in definitive repair require careful monitoring and control of the patient's blood pressure in the intensive care unit, using beta blockers, nitrates, or both, as required.

When diagnosed, operative repair should be performed as soon as possible. This most often entails tube graft replacement of the involved infrarenal aorta, similar to the repair of an abdominal aortic aneurysm. Much less frequently, the injury may be managed by suturing an intimal flap or thromboendarterectomy. Catheter embolectomy of the lower extremities should be performed routinely at the completion of the repair in all cases of traumatic thrombosis, because peripheral embolization has been reported as a complication in 35% of cases in this setting.

Indications for limited delay in repair of stable injuries in the absence of distal ischemia may include concomitant head injury (where heparin is contraindicated), and instances of gross gastrointestinal contamination where extra-anatomic bypass would otherwise be required.

Injuries to the Portal Venous System

Although uncommon, injuries to the portal venous system may present some of the more difficult management problems in abdominal trauma. The overwhelming majority of these injuries are secondary to penetrating trauma, primarily gunshot wounds. Reported mortality rates range between 35 and 45% overall, and are considerably higher for injury involving the portal vein (50 to 70%).[47–50] The high mortality rate for portal vein injury is attributed primarily to associated major vascular injuries, as well as the difficulty of rapidly gaining adequate exposure, particularly for injury to the retropancreatic segment (Fig. 11–5). Nearly 100% of patients with portal vein injury have concomitant injuries to adjacent organs, and 70% have injury to an adjacent major vascular structure.[48,49] In decreasing order, the most frequently associated vascular injuries include vena cava, aorta, and superior mesenteric artery.[48,49,51] In many cases, management of the associated vascular injury may take priority over definitive repair of the portal venous injury.

Initial control of bleeding from a suprapancreatic portal venous injury may often be obtained by performing a Pringle maneuver, inserting the index finger into the foramen of Winslow and compressing the porta structures against the thumb.[49] An adjunctive measure for control of portal vein injuries in the region of the hilum is intraluminal occlusion via passage of a Fogarty balloon catheter.[51] Vigorous venous bleeding from injuries below the hepatoduodenal ligament, often associated with an injury to the head of the pancreas, is best controlled temporarily with laparotomy packs and direct pressure until better exposure can be obtained.

Several techniques are useful in achieving maximal exposure for injuries of the portal venous system. The lateral peritoneal reflection or hepatic flexure is divided, reflecting the right colon and small bowel mesentery medially. The duodenum and head of the pancreas should be mobilized medially via a generous Kocher maneuver. Dissection of the plane between the duodenum and small bowel mesentery provides good exposure of the superior mesenteric vein.

Injuries of the suprapancreatic portal vein are exposed by further dissection of

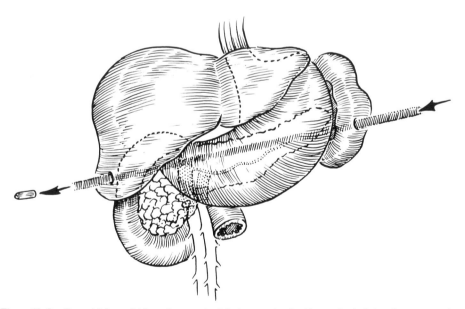

Figure 11–5. Potential for multiple major vascular injuries associated with portal vein injury from penetrating trauma.

structures in the porta. The common bile duct is mobilized anteriorly and laterally, using vascular loops to provide gentle traction. Exposure of injuries near the hilum is augmented by division of the cystic duct, with subsequent cholecystectomy to be performed after repair of the vascular injuries.[47,48]

Exposure and control of an injury to the retropancreatic portal vein may be considerably more difficult. Stone et al[49] reported a 100% mortality rate for injuries at the confluence of the portal vein and superior mesenteric vein. Injuries to this region are exposed by division of the neck of the pancreas after first mobilizing the hepatic flexure and small bowel, as described previously. In some cases, this may simply complete a transection already begun by the initial injury. The distal pancreas is later managed by internal drainage or distal pancreatectomy, depending on the condition of the patient and associated injuries. An additional maneuver that may be useful is mobilization of the spleen and tail of the pancreas medially, approaching the portal vein from the left. This allows the splenic vein to act as a "handle," assisting in exposure of an injury in this location.

Definitive management of injuries to the portal vein most frequently entails primary lateral venorrhaphy.[47–49,51] For treatment of more severe injuries, several complex reconstructive procedures have been described, including end-to-end reanastomosis, segmental interposition grafting, transposition of the splenic vein to the superior mesenteric vein, and portosystemic shunting.[52] These procedures were used at a time when it was believed that ligation of the portal vein should be avoided at all costs, out of fear of mesenteric venous infarction, development of portal venous hypertension, and venous pooling in the splancnic circulation resulting in severe hypovolemia. Previously, a 100% mortality rate had been reported for acute portal vein ligation in dog studies.[52] The above procedures are, under optimal circumstances, difficult to perform, and this is compounded by the hypothermia and coagulopathy often encountered in patients sustaining these severe injuries. Additionally, postsystemic shunting in patients with previously normal hepatic circulation may be expected to cause severe encephalopathy and result in high postoperative mortality.[49,50,53,54]

Further experience has shown that ligation of the portal vein is the treatment of choice for complex injuries that cannot be managed by lateral repair. Stone et al[49] have demonstrated an 80% long-term survival for severe injuries of the portal vein treated by simple ligation. They and others accurately emphasize that the chief pitfall to be encountered within the first 72 hours after portal vein ligation is significant splancnic venous pooling, which occurs at the expense of profound peripheral hypovolemia.[49,52] The two deaths that occurred in the Stone et al series were attributed to this problem, with inadequate replacement of peripheral fluid volume postoperatively. Aggressive volume resuscitation therefore must be continued for the first 24 to 72 hours postoperatively in patients undergoing ligation of the portal vein. Adequacy of fluid or blood replacement in this setting is best determined by right heart catheterization. Fears of portal hypertension postoperatively so far have not been realized. Five of eight survivors in the Stone et al series underwent angiography 2 months to 3 years after operation. All were noted to have developed excellent venous collateralization to the liver, with no evidence of residual portal hypertension.[49] Venous infarction of the bowel has also not been observed in several series of patients undergoing portal or superior mesenteric venous ligation for trauma.[48,49,51]

An exception to the above rule occurs when a concomitant hepatic artery injury exists. In this circumstance, at least one of these vessels must be reliably reconstructed to avoid hepatic necrosis and death.

Injuries of the superior mesenteric vein are handled similarly to the portal vein. Overall reported mortality rates are less than in portal vein injuries, because of easier exposure and a lower incidence of associated major vascular injuries.[49] The treatment of choice is primary lateral venorrhaphy, with ligation reserved for more complex defects. Survival following ligation is reported to be between 67 and 90%.[48,49] As in portal vein ligation, aggressive postoperative volume replacement is required.

Most injuries of the splenic and inferior mesenteric veins may be ligated safely if lateral repair is not easily accomplished. Splenic vein ligation should be followed by splenectomy to avoid the possibility of splenic infarction postoperatively.[48]

Renovascular Injuries

Vascular injuries to the renal artery, vein, or both, are relatively uncommon, with large series being reported only over a long period of time and from the busiest urban trauma centers. Reported mortality rates range from 12% to 39%, and are attributed primarily to associated injuries.[55–57] Regardless of mechanism of injury, a nearly 100% incidence of associated intra-abdominal injury is reported, with several large reviews reporting an average of over three associated injuries per patient.[55–58] The number and severity of associated injuries, therefore, may have an important role in management decisions regarding renovascular injury. For example, an unstable patient with severe concomitant injuries and a normally functioning contralateral kidney would not be a candidate for a complex vascular repair; in this case nephrectomy is a more appropriate form of management. The majority of renovascular injuries are of penetrating etiology, primarily gunshot wounds, followed by stab wounds and shotgun wounds.[59] Blunt injuries requiring surgical intervention are, in general, less common and are more frequently accompanied by a significant delay in diagnosis. The overwhelming majority of these are secondary to motor vehicle crashes. For reasons that are not entirely clear, the left renal artery is injured more frequently than the right in blunt trauma.[60,61] Proposed mechanisms of renal artery injury in blunt trauma include severe deceleration, in which the relatively mobile kidney causes stretching of the renal artery with intimal disruption and subsequent thrombosis. A second possible mechanism involves compression of the artery between the anterior abdominal wall and vertebral column, such as might occur with a steering wheel injury, resulting in severe contusion and thrombosis.[52]

Prompt diagnosis is essential if surgical repair of a renovascular injury for renal salvage is to be successful. Urinalysis is notoriously unreliable; 28 to 36% of patients with significant vascular injury to the renal pedicle may present without even microscopic hematuria.[61,62] Likewise, urine output is of little use, because this may be sustained by the output of the contralateral kidney. Intravenous pyelography (IVP) remains the single best screening test to evaluate for vascular injury to the renal pedicle and should, when possible, be performed on all patients undergoing celiotomy for abdominal trauma.[63] Additional indications for urgent IVP include gross or microscopic hematuria and persistent flank or abdominal pain in patients having sustained blunt abdominal trauma.[62]

Visualization of both kidneys on a 3-minute "one-shot" IVP provides the knowledge that significant renal vascular injury is unlikely and, if an unexpected injury is discovered at subsequent celiotomy, there is a functional contralateral kidney. Intravenous contrast medium given at the time of abdominal computed tomography (CT) scanning can provide similar information as well as additional anatomic detail. Nonvisualization of a kidney on IVP is not, however, an absolute indication of arterial thrombosis. In a recent review, Cass et al[61] found that of 52 nonfunctioning kidneys on IVP, only 21 were found at arteriography or exploration to have arterial thrombosis. Other causes of nonvisualization on IVP may include vasospasm, severe hypovolemia, contusion, rupture, or laceration. In patients whose condition permits therefore, a nonfunctioning kidney on IVP is an indication for immediate arteriography to confirm the diagnosis and define the injury.[57] An aortogram is usually adequate to visualize the renal arteries in most patients and can avoid the added time and morbidity of selective renal arteriography.[63] Radionuclide imaging may confirm the diagnosis of vascular injury; however, this does not provide adequate detail to define the injury if operative intervention is planned.

Management of vascular injuries to the renal pedicle depends on the mechanism of injury, delay between injury and diagnosis, associated injuries, and condition of the patient. Penetrating injuries most frequently come to celiotomy with minimal delay because of the high likelihood of major concomitant abdominal injuries. Findings at celiotomy will usually include a perirenal or midline hematoma, which may or may not be expanding. In general, all such hematomas should be explored. Proximal vascular control is mandatory before exploration.[55] Isolation of the renal vasculature may be accomplished via a midline approach. The transverse mesocolon is retracted superiorly and duodenum and small bowel retracted to the right. The peritoneum anterior to the aorta is incised vertically and the fourth portion of the duodenum mobilized gently toward the right. The dissection is carried superiorly on the anterior wall of the aorta until the left renal vein is encountered. The vessel is mobilized carefully and isolated with a Rumel tourniquet, which can be used to provide gentle traction. Retracting the vein anteriorly and superiorly, the dissection is continued upward until the takeoff of the left renal artery is identified. This, too, is encircled with a Rumel tourniquet to provide proximal control. The right renal artery is identified and controlled in a similar fashion. The right renal vein may be more difficult to expose from this approach and requires further dissection toward the right, anterior to the vena cava.[55] A technically simpler approach to the right renal vein, which may risk violating the hematoma before control is obtained, involves exposure via a Kocher maneuver, mobilizing the duodenum and head of the pancreas toward the left. The renal vein may then be isolated under direct vision near its confluence with the vena cava. It should be remembered that in patients found to have a midline hematoma a significant possibility exists of an aortic injury.[55,57] Before any attempt to expose the renal pedicles therefore, proximal control of the aorta should be obtained, as described previously for injuries to the suprarenal aorta.

Operative management of penetrating injuries brought promptly to exploration depends on the complexity of the injury and condition of the patient. Extended attempts at renal revascularization in a patient with severe concomitant injuries and a functional contralateral kidney are unwarranted.[55,61] Simple lacerations of the artery or vein are best managed by lateral repair using 5-0 polypropylene vascular suture. Larger defects may require segmental resection, followed by end-to-end reanastomosis, interposition grafting, or aortorenal bypass, as required. Occasionally, revascularization may be accomplished using splenic artery or inferior mesenteric artery.[55] Injuries requiring more complex procedures than lateral repair are associated with a significantly higher secondary nephrectomy rate (65% compared with 15% for lateral repair in large series reported by Brown et al[55]), which should be considered when deciding whether to revascularize. Prolonged warm ischemia time probably contributes significantly to this increased failure rate; useful adjunctive measures to alleviate this may include perfusion of the injured kidney with cold lactated Ringer's solution using a small balloon catheter, local packing with ice in laparotomy packs, or both. Injuries to the left renal vein may be treated safely by ligation without nephrectomy, provided collateral drainage via the gonadal or adrenal veins is preserved. Right renal vein injuries requiring ligation are best treated by nephrectomy because of inadequate collateral drainage.[3] Severe blast injuries to the hilum and complex injuries involving both the renal artery and vein should be treated by nephrectomy rather than an attempt at repair.[55]

Appropriate management of blunt injuries to the renal pedicle is less clear-cut and somewhat controversial. Originally described by Von Recklinghausen in 1861,[64] this injury is seen infrequently, but is no longer considered rare. Results of attempted renal salvage for blunt trauma are, in general, dismal, primarily because of frequent delays in diagnosis and resultant prolonged warm ischemia time. Diagnostic delay may result from minimal symptoms, altered mental status caused by concomitant head injury or intoxication, or the presence of more life-threatening injuries.

The decision to explore and attempt revascularization for a unilateral blunt renovascular injury hinges on the condition of the patient and period of time between injury and diagnosis. Classically, it is believed that normal kidneys will tolerate only 1 to 2 hours of warm ischemia time before irreversible damage occurs.[65,66] Clinical experience with traumatic injuries has shown that in some cases 12 to 18 hours of ischemia may be tolerated with at least partial return of renal function on revascularization.[58,62,63] It is important to point out, however, that in unilateral injury successful renal salvage implies not only documented return of function, but also absence of persistent hypertension leading to delayed nephrectomy.

Given the above criteria, successful renal salvage may be accomplished in approximately 15 to 35% of those attempted.[58,63] Successful outcome after more than 18 hours is highly unusual. Postoperatively, a successfully revascularized kidney may be expected to recover slowly; return of function may require 6 to 8 weeks or longer.[62] Long-term success may be documented without toxicity by serial ultrasound examination and radionuclide scanning.

Although the above results are far from ideal, they are superior to the 100% loss of function that may be expected if revascularization is not attempted.[61] In a young, stable, good-risk patient in whom the diagnosis is made promptly therefore, revascularization of unilateral blunt renal artery thrombosis should be attempted.[61,63]

It should also be emphasized that the dismal statistics apply primarily to injuries involving complete thrombosis or avulsion of the renal artery; patients displaying opacification of the distal renal vessels or partial occlusion of the main artery by an intimal flap demonstrate a considerably better operative success rate.[67] Reduced perfusion of the kidney in this setting may prevent effective function, yet allow for continued viability and therefore a potentially salvageable organ.[68,69] This may occur even after the usually terminal 18-hour postinjury period. Thus, in this setting the period after injury for which revascularization is a consideration may be extended indefinitely.[68]

Bilateral renal artery thrombosis from blunt trauma is a rare, but occasionally reported, injury. Indications for attempted revascularization for this injury may be extended for as long as 48 to 72 hours postinjury; any return of renal function that might spare the patient permanent hemodialysis justifies the added morbidity of operation in all but poor-risk patients.[58] This aggressive policy applies equally to patients with solitary kidneys because of unilateral renal agenesis or previous nephrectomy.

Operative management of blunt renal artery thrombosis requires reconstruction via bypass, excision and reanastomosis, or patch angioplasty after initial thrombectomy; simple thrombectomy alone is inadequate and will result in recurrent thrombosis because of the underlying intimal injury.[63]

In patients in whom an infarcted kidney is diagnosed, those not candidates for revascularization, and those who do not require exploration for other indications, little is to be gained by early nephrectomy.[63] Less than half of these patients will ultimately develop complications requiring later nephrectomy. Indications for delayed nephrectomy include persistent hypertension, pain from renal infarction, and infectious complications.

Perinephric hematomas may be encountered in blunt injury where the patient has undergone celiotomy for unrelated blunt injuries. Those that are nonexpanding and in which preoperative or intraoperative IVP visualizes both kidneys need not be explored for vascular indications.[61] Expanding hematomas or failure to visualize the kidney on IVP demands exploration. Nephrectomy or revascularization may then be performed, depending on the condition of the patient and length of previous ischemia time.

Vascular Injuries to the Pelvis

Vascular injuries in the pelvis can be divided into the two common etiologic categories: penetrating and blunt, which require distinctly different modes of management.

Vascular injuries to the pelvis as a result of penetrating trauma are caused primarily by gunshot wounds, followed by shotgun and stab wounds in decreasing order of frequency. Penetrating injuries to the iliac vessels carry a reported mortality rate of 25 to 52%.[70-72] This is attributed to the difficulty of rapidly gaining control of injured vessels deep in the pelvis and a high incidence of free hemorrhage into the peritoneal cavity rather than tamponade. Ryan et al[70] reported a 46% incidence of active hemorrhage into the peritoneal cavity at the time of operation for injuries to the iliac vessels; free hemorrhage was associated with a 46% mortality rate compared with 93% survival for injuries with an intact tamponade. Associated intra-abdominal injuries are common (89 to 95%) and in decreasing order of frequency include small bowel, colon, ureter, and bladder.[70-72]

Preoperative evaluation is minimal because most patients have hypotension (52 to 82%) and a penetrating injury, most commonly below the umbilicus. The clinical triad of hypotension, positive abdominal findings, and a penetrating injury below the umbilicus was present in 76% of patients in a recent series of 114 patients.[70] Peripheral pulse deficits are less common (25 to 39%), but are diagnostic of arterial injury.[70-72] After appropriate resuscitative measures, the patient should be brought to celiotomy without delay.

Operative management initially centers on rapid control of ongoing hemorrhage. Active hemorrhage into the peritoneal cavity from within the pelvis is best handled initially by direct packing of the bleeding site with manual pressure. This may be followed by cross-clamping the aorta below the renal arteries. Manual pressure at the pelvic brim and groin may also help to achieve temporary control while the area of the injury is dissected further and isolated.

Operative management of penetrating injuries to the iliac vessels most often entails lateral repair or resection of the injured portion with primary end-to-end reanastomosis.[70–72] Severe injury to the internal iliac vessels may be managed safely by ligation. Occasionally, large defects in the common or external iliac vessels may require interposition grafting, using prosthetic material, saphenous vein, or hypogastric artery. The risk of septic complications is significant because of frequent concomitant gastrointestinal injuries. Millikan et al[72] therefore recommend the use of prosthetic material only in injuries not associated with violation of the gastrointestinal tract. Mattox et al[71] point out that a Dacron graft infection results in an anastomotic leak, pseudoaneurysm formation, or both, while an infected autogenous graft results in complete dissolution of the graft with massive and potentially fatal hemorrhage. They believe therefore that the higher infection rate with Dacron grafts (three of six in their series) is acceptable, because the complication can be successfully managed (three of three) by graft resection, ligation, and extra-anatomic bypass if required. This topic remains controversial.

In injuries where severe contamination may preclude the use of graft material in the operative field, extra-anatomic bypass via the femorofemoral route as the initial operative management is also an acceptable alternative. It should also be remembered that in patients who are unstable, have developed hypothermia or coagulopathy, or have life-threatening concomitant injuries, simple ligation of the common or external iliac artery may be the most appropriate management; prolonged attempts at reconstruction in this setting may result in a revascularized limb and dead patient.

Venous injuries should, as well, be repaired when feasible.[73,74] Sequelae of major vein ligation may include chronic edema, skin breakdown, and failure of arterial reconstruction resulting in amputation. The primary difficulty in managing injuries to the iliac veins is in obtaining adequate exposure. As described earlier in this chapter, division of the common iliac artery may occasionally be required to gain exposure of the proximal common iliac vein, located posteriorly; the artery is then repaired primarily.[42] Similarly, for exposure of venous injuries located more distally, the hypogastric artery may be divided and mobilized to improve exposure and does not require subsequent repair.[75]

Bleeding from severe soft tissue injuries, such as from a shotgun or high-velocity missile wounds, may result in severe diffuse venous bleeding even in the absence of injury to named vascular structures. Prolonged efforts at suture ligation of multiple small bleeding sites in this situation may prove futile. In selected patients therefore firm packing with laparotomy packs and planned reoperation for their removal may be more appropriate, similar to the management of major liver injuries.

Occasional iatrogenic injuries to the iliac vessels may occur as a result of attempts at percutaneous transcatheter dilation of atherosclerotic lesions, placement of internal fixation screws during hip arthroplasty, and during lumbar laminectomy. Hemorrhage from a perforation of the external or common iliac vessels as a result of balloon angioplasty may be controlled by occlusion of the vessel intraluminally with steel coils, if the injury is recognized at the time of the procedure when the catheter is still in place.[76,77] Alternatively, the perforation may be temporarily occluded with an angioplasty balloon catheter.[78] The patient is then brought to the operating room for definitive treatment. If hemorrhage has been successfully controlled with coils, revascularization of the involved side is carried out by aortofemoral bypass or extra-anatomic route, depending on the condition of the patient. If the injury has been temporarily occluded by the balloon, it may be approached via retroperitoneal dissection for repair via thrombectomy and patch angioplasty.[78]

Injury to the external iliac vessels from placement of acetabular screws during an orthopedic procedure may result in acute hemodynamic instability of the patient on the operating table. This can indicate decompression of the vascular injury into the peritoneal cavity and should be managed by immediate celiotomy. Operative treatment proceeds as for penetrating injuries, as previously described. Injury of the artery may also present as thrombosis postoperatively, manifested by acute extremity ischemia, loss of peripheral pulses, and lower quadrant abdominal pain if extravasation has occurred. The diagnosis is then confirmed via emergent aortography, followed by repair via retroperitoneal approach.[79] This may entail thrombectomy followed by patch angioplasty or interposition grafting. Inadvertent injury to the proximal iliac vessels during lumbar laminectomy will result in a large hematoma posteriorly and are best approached anteriorly via celiotomy, which allows rapid control of the infrarenal aorta and contralateral iliac vessels. Management is then the same as for any penetrating injury in this region.

As alluded to in the beginning of this chapter, management of retroperitoneal hemorrhage from blunt injuries is primarily nonoperative. Early mortality in severe pelvic fractures is mainly attributed to failure to control retroperitoneal blood loss in the pelvis and frequent concomitant neurologic injury.[7] Mortality rates for those patients with hemodynamic instability is reported to be 42%, compared with 3% for those not presenting in shock.[6] A mortality rate of 50% or more is associated with open pelvic fracture, where the beneficial effect of retroperitoneal tamponade is lost. Results of attempted direct operative control of hemorrhage in this setting, usually via hypogastric artery ligation, suture ligature of individual bleeders, or attempts at intraoperative embolization, have been exceedingly poor.[6,10,17] The rich arterial and venous collateral circulation in the pelvis prevent ligation of proximal arterial vessels from being an effective form of therapy. When exploration is required for concomitant injuries, every effort should be made to avoid violation of the pelvic retroperitoneal hematoma, because this can release a tamponade, resulting in massive and uncontrollable hemorrhage.

SUMMARY

Retroperitoneal vascular injuries are predominantly penetrating in etiology and carry a high mortality rate. The high hospital mortality reflects not only the magnitude of the vascular injury, but also the severity and frequency of associated organ injuries. Retroperitoneal vascular injuries secondary to blunt trauma are associated with pelvic fractures in the vast majority of cases.

Survivors of major vascular injuries in the retroperitoneum have contained retroperitoneal hematomas in almost all cases. If the vascular injury is not tamponaded by the retroperitoneum, and free hemorrhage into the abdominal cavity is present, mortality is extremely high. Therefore, the surgeon is most often confronted in the operating room by a contained retroperitoneal hematoma. In blunt trauma, the approach to these retroperitoneal hematomas is dictated by the zone in which the hematomas are located. The lateral retroperitoneal hematomas are most commonly associated with renal injuries and are only entered if appropriate indications are met. Pelvic hematomas are almost exclusively associated with pelvic fractures, and these hematomas are left intact, almost without exception. Retroperitoneal hematomas in the central zone must be entered and explored due to the high incidence of major vascular injury. These hematomas are entered only after proximal and distal vascular control has been appropriately obtained. By following the basic tenets of good vascular surgery, with appropriate vascular control, excellent survivability can be achieved in vena cava, aortic, and renal vascular injuries. Retrohepatic venous or vena caval injuries continue to carry an extremely high mortality secondary to the difficulty in obtaining adequate exposure and vascular control.

Retroperitoneal hematomas secondary to penetrating injuries all must be explored. Again, the hematoma should only be entered after appropriate vascular control has been obtained. Patient salvage can be excellent with a contained retroperitoneal hematoma and proper operative strategy.

Hemorrhage control associated with pelvic fracture depends on rapid recognition of the pelvic fracture, its potential for exsanguinating hemorrhage, and immediate institution of appropriate therapy. Fracture stabilization with Military Antishock Trousers garment and external fixators and early arteriography with embolization will aid in decreasing the mortality of these high energy injuries.

REFERENCES

1. Weil PH: Management of retroperitoneal trauma. *Curr Prob Surg* 1983;49:540–621.
2. Weincek RG, Wilson RF: Injuries to the abdominal vascular system: How much does aggressive resuscitation and prelaparotomy thoractomy really help? *Surgery* 1983;102:731–736.
3. Feliciano DV: Abdominal vascular injuries. *Surg Clin North Am* 1988;68:741–755.
4. Kashuk JL, Moore EE, Millikan MD, et al: Major abdominal vascular trauma—a unified approach. *J Trauma* 1982;22:672–679.
5. Thal ER, McClelland RN, Shires GT: Abdominal trauma. In Shires GT (ed): *Trauma Care*, 3rd ed. New York: McGraw-Hill Book Co., 1986, pp 291–344.
6. Mucha P Jr, Welch TJ: Hemorrhage in major pelvic fractures. *Surg Clin North Am* 1988;68:757–773.
7. Rothenberger DA, Fisher RP, Strate RG, et al: The mortality associated with pelvic fractures. *Surgery* 1978;84:356–361.
8. Binder SS, Mitchell GA: Control of intractable pelvic hemorrhage by ligation of the hypogastric artery. *South Med J* 1960;53:837–843.
9. Hauser CW, Perry JF Jr: Control of massive hemorrhage from pelvic fractures by hypogastric artery ligation. *Surg Gynecol Obstet* 1965;121:313–315.
10. Ravitch MM: Hypogastric artery ligation in acute pelvic trauma. *Surgery* 1964;56:601–602.
11. Feliciano DV, Bitondo CG, Cruse PA, et al: Liberal use of emergency center thoracotomy. *Am J Surg* 1986;152:654–659.
12. Moore EE, Moore JB, Galloway AC, et al: Post-injury thoracotomy in the emergency department: A critical evaluation. *Surgery* 1979;86:590–598.
13. Weincek RG, Wilson RF: Abdominal venous injuries. *J Trauma* 1986;26:771–778.
14. Gilliland MG, Ward RG, Flynn TC, et al: Peritoneal lavage and angiography in the management of patients with pelvic fractures. *Am J Surg* 1982;144:744–747.
15. Panetta T, Scalfani SJA, Goldstein AS, et al: Percutaneous transcatheter embolization for massive bleeding from pelvic fractures. *J Trauma* 1985;25:1021–1029.
16. Hubbard SG, Bivins BA, Schatello CR, et al: Diagnostic errors with peritoneal lavage in patients with pelvic fractures. *Arch Surg* 1979;144:844–846.
17. Flint LM, Brown A, Richardson JD, et al: Definitive control of bleeding from severe pelvic fractures. *Ann Surg* 1979;189:709–716.
18. Moreno C, Moore EE, Rosenberger A, et al: Hemorrhage associated with major pelvic fracture: A multispecialty challenge. *J Trauma* 1986;26:987–994.
19. Posner CM, Moore EE, Greenholz MD, et al: Natural history of untreated inferior vena cava injury and assessment of venous access. *J Trauma* 1986;26:698–701.
20. Stewart MT, Stone HH: Injuries of the inferior vena cava. *Am Surg* 1986;52:9–13.
21. Burch JM, Feliciano DV, Mattox KL: The atriocaval shunt: Facts and fiction. *Ann Surg* 1988;207:555–568.
22. Weincek RG Jr, Wilson RF: Inferior vena cava injuries: The challenge continues. *Am Surg* 1988;54:423–428.
23. Turpin I, State D, Schwartz A: Injuries to the vena cava and their management. *Am J Surg* 1977;134:25–32.
24. Bricker DL, Morton JR, Okies JE, et al: Surgical management of injuries to the vena cava: Changing patterns of injury and newer techniques of repair. *J Trauma* 1971;11:725–735.

25. James EC, Fedde CW, Khuri NT, et al: Division of the left renal vein: A safe surgical adjunct. *Surgery* 1978;83:151–154.
26. Misra B, Wagner R, Boneval H: Injuries of the hepatic veins and retrohepatic cava. *Am Surg* 1983;49:55–60.
27. Schrock T, Blaisdell FW, Mathewson CJ Jr: Management of blunt trauma to the liver and hepatic veins. *Arch Surg* 1968;96:698–704.
28. Yellin AE, Chaffee CB, Donovan AJ: Vascular isolation in treatment of juxtahepatic venous injuries. *Arch Surg* 1971;102:566–573.
29. Rovita PF: Atrio caval shunting in blunt hepatic vascular injury. *Ann Surg* 1987;205:318–321.
30. Heaney JP, Jacobsen A: Simplified control of upper abdominal hemorrhage from the vena cava. *Surgery* 1975;78:138–141.
31. Pilcher BP, Harman PK, Moore EE: Retrohepatic vena cava balloon shunt introduced via the saphenofemoral junction. *J Trauma* 1977;17:837–841.
32. Pachter HL, Spencer FC, Hofstetter SR, et al: The management of juxtahepatic venous injuries without an atriocaval shunt: Preliminary clinical observations. *Surgery* 1986;99:569–575.
33. Depinto LD, Mucha SJ, Powers PC: Major hepatic vein ligation necessitated by blunt trauma. *Ann Surg* 1976;183:243–246.
34. Frame SB, Timberlake GA, Rush DS, et al: Penetrating injuries of the abdominal aorta. *Am Surg* 1990;56:651–654.
35. Brinton M, Miller SE, Lim RC, et al: Acute abdominal aortic injuries. *J Trauma* 1982;22:481–486.
36. Millikan JS, Moore EE: Critical factors in determining mortality from abdominal aortic trauma. *Surg Gynecol Obstet* 1985;160:313–316.
37. Mattox KL, Burch JM, Richardson R, et al: Retroperitoneal vascular injury. *Surg Clin North Am* 1990;70:635–653.
38. Mattox KL, McCollum WB, Jordan GL, et al: Management of upper abdominal vascular trauma. *Am J Surg* 1974;128:823–828.
39. Accola KD, Feliciano DV, Mattox KL, et al: Management of injuries to the suprarenal aorta. *Am J Surg* 1987;154:613–618.
40. Mattox KL, Whisenand HH, Beall AC, et al: Management of acute combined injuries to the aorta and inferior vena cava. *Am J Surg* 1975;130:720–724.
41. Mattox KL, McCullum KB, Beall AC, et al: Management of penetrating injuries of the suprarenal aorta. *J Trauma* 1975;15:808–815.
42. Salam AA, Stewart MT: A new approach to wounds of the aortic bifurcation and vena cava. *Surgery* 1985;98:105–108.
43. Lassonde J, Laurendeau F: Blunt injury of the abdominal aorta. *Ann Surg* 1981;194:745–748.
44. Lock JS, Huffman AD, Johnson RC: Blunt trauma to the abdominal aorta. *J Trauma* 1987;27:674–677.
45. Parmley LF, Mattingly TW, Manion WC, et al: Nonpenetrating traumatic injury of the aorta. *Circulation* 1958;17:1086–1101.
46. Strassman G: Traumatic rupture of the aorta. *Am J Heart* 1947;33:508–515.
47. Sheldon GF, Lim RC, Yee ES, et al: Management of injuries to the porta hepatis. *Ann Surg* 1985;202:539–545.
48. Graham JM, Mattox KL, Beall AC: Portal venous system injuries. *J Trauma* 1978;18:419–422.
49. Stone IIII, Fabian TC, Turkleson ML: Wounds of the portal venous system. *World J Surg* 1982;6:335–341.
50. Dawson DL, Johansen KH, Jurkovich GJ: Injuries to the portal triad. *Am J Surg* 1991;161:545–551.
51. Petersen SR, Sheldon GF, Lim RC: Management of portal vein injuries. *J Trauma* 1979;19:616–620.
52. Busuttil RW, Kitahama A, Cerise E, et al: Management of blunt and penetrating injuries to the porta hepatis. *Ann Surg* 1980;191:641–648.
53. Fish JC: Reconstruction of the portal vein. Case reports and literature review. *Am Surg* 1966;32:472–478.
54. Malt RA: Portosystemic venous shunts. Part I. *N Engl J Med* 1976;295:24–29.
55. Brown MF, Graham JM, Mattox KL, et al: Renovascular trauma. *Am J Surg* 1980;140:802–805.
56. Meacham PW, Brock JW, Kirchner FK, et al: Renal vascular injuries. *Am Surg* 1985;52:30–36.
57. Sagalowsky AI, McDonnell JD, Peters PC: Renal trauma requiring surgery: An analysis of 185 cases. *J Trauma* 1983;23:128–131.
58. Sprinak JP, Resnick MI: Revascularization of traumatic thrombosis of the renal artery. *Surg Gynecol Obstet* 1987;164:22–26.
59. Carroll PR, McAninch JW, Klosterman P, et al: Renovascular trauma: Risk assessment, surgical management, and outcome. *J Trauma* 1990;30:547–554.
60. Maggio AJ, Brosman S: Renal artery trauma. *Urology* 1978;11:125–130.
61. Cass AS, Bubrick M, Luxenberg M, et al: Renal pedicle injury in patients with multiple injuries. *J Trauma* 1985;25:892–896.
62. Barlow B, Gandhi R: Renal artery thrombosis following blunt trauma. *J Trauma* 1980;20:614–617.
63. Clark DE, Georgitis JW, Ray FS: Renal arterial injuries caused by blunt trauma. *J Trauma* 1981;90:87–96.
64. Von Recklinghausen F: Hemorrhagishe niereninfarkte. *Virchows Arch Pathol Anat* 1861;20:205.

65. Magilligan DJ, DeWeese JA, May AG, et al: The occluded renal artery. *Surgery* 1975;78:730–736.
66. Vollmar J, Helmstadler D, Hallwachs O: Complete occlusion of the renal artery: Nephrectomy or revascularization? *J Cardiovasc Surg* 1971;12:441–446.
67. Turner WW, Snyder WH, Fry WJ: Mortality and renal salvage after renovascular trauma. *Am J Surg* 1983;146:848–851.
68. Greeholz SK, Moore EE, Peterson NE, et al: Traumatic bilateral renal artery occlusion: Successful outcome without surgical intervention. *J Trauma* 1986;26:941–944.
69. Dean RH: Management of renal artery trauma. (Editorial.) *J Vasc Surg* 1988;8:89–90.
70. Ryan W, Snyder W, Bell T, et al: Penetrating injuries of the iliac vessels. *Am J Surg* 1982;144:642–645.
71. Mattox KL, Rea J, Ennix CL, et al: Penetrating injuries to the iliac arteries. *Am J Surg* 1978;136:663–667.
72. Millikan JS, Moore EE, Van Way CW, et al: Vascular trauma in the groin: Contrast between iliac and femoral injuries. *Am J Surg* 1981;142:695–698.
73. Rich NM, Collins GJ, Andersen CA, et al: Venous trauma; Successful venous reconstruction remains an interesting challenge. *Am J Surg* 1977;134:226–230.
74. Rich NM, Andersen CA, McDonald PT: Autogenous venous interposition grafts in repair of major venous injuries. *J Trauma* 1977;17:512–520.
75. Vitelli CE, Scalea TM, Philips TF, et al: A technique for controlling injuries of the iliac vein in the patient with trauma. *Surg Gynecol Obstet* 1988;166:551–552.
76. Jensen SR, Voegeli DR, Crummy AB, et al: Iliac artery rupture during transluminal angioplasty: Treatment by embolization and surgical bypass. *AJR* 1985;145:381–382.
77. Simonetti G, Rossi P, Passariello R, et al: Iliac artery rupture: A complication of transluminal angioplasty. *AJR* 1983;140:989–990.
78. Villarica J, Gross RC: Treatment of angioplasty related iliac artery rupture without bypass surgery (case report). *AJR* 1986;147:389–390.
79. Jonsson H Jr, Karlstrom G, Lundovist B: Intimal rupture and arterial thrombosis in revisional hip arthroplasty. *Acta Chi Scand* 1987;153:621–622.

12

Genitourinary Tract Trauma

SCOTT B. FRAME, M.D., F.A.C.S.

The renal system consists of paired kidneys lying in the lateral retroperitoneum, paired ureters carrying urine from the kidneys to the single, midline bladder lying in the pelvis, and the urethra, present to permit the passage of urine to the outside world. These structures lie in a relatively protected environment, but injuries are still present in 10 to 15% of all abdominal trauma.[1-3] Blunt trauma accounts for approximately 80% of all renal injuries.[3] The same, remote, anatomic location that affords some protection to these structures makes the early diagnosis of injuries difficult. Delayed diagnosis may lead to a multitude of complications, such as: bleeding, urinary extravasation, infection, abscess formation, and loss of body parts.

The earliest documentation in the literature of an injury to the urinary system may be found in Homer's *Iliad*.[4] In this classic of literature, the "spear of Merion" is said to have pierced the urinary bladder and caused a fatal injury. Galen and Hippocrates also cited deaths from urinary bladder injuries.[4] The first to advocate urinary diversion for the treatment of bladder injuries was Chopart in 1792.[5] In 1905, Evans and Fowler[6] described laparotomy, evacuation of urine, and closure of intraperitoneal bladder injuries. This method of treatment was shown to reduce the mortality of these injuries from 100 to 28%. Suprapubic drainage of bladder injuries was first described in 1936 by Hinman,[7] and remains the method of choice for bladder diversion to this day.

Ambroise Paré[8] is credited with the first description of a renal wound secondary to gunshot. In 1585 Paré published *The Apologie and Treatise*, in which is described his voyage of Hedin in 1553. Paré reports on the gunshot wound of Monsieur de Martigues. The bullet entered the chest and was noted to travel into the abdomen. The patient is described as passing copious amounts of blood in his urine during the several days prior to his death. Unfortunately, Paré did not correlate the hematuria with injury to the kidney.

DIAGNOSIS

Patient History

The approach to the diagnosis of injuries to the urinary system follows the same tenets as the diagnosis of any malady in medicine. Halsteadian philosophy maintains that the history

157

represents 90% of the diagnosis. This follows in trauma and holds true in renal injuries. A careful history of the traumatic event will yield those patients who are at risk for urinary system trauma.

High-speed decelerations, as occur in head-on motor vehicle accidents, falls from heights, and motor vehicle–pedestrian accidents, are associated with renal pedicle and parenchymal injuries. Assaults and contact sports are also known to result in renal trauma. Blows to the flank by blunt objects should be thoroughly investigated. Any patient with trauma to the back, flanks, abdomen, or lower chest severe enough to cause a skin contusion may have renal trauma, regardless of whether symptoms are present or not. Sharp blows to the abdomen in the presence of a full bladder may result in bladder rupture, in the absence of a pelvic fracture.

In penetrating trauma, the caliber of the gun and distance from which the shot was fired are valuable pieces of information to obtain. These data will yield information on the potential tissue destruction that might be expected. The size and type of sharp instrument used in stab wounds may aid in planning the diagnostic scheme to be followed in determining urinary injury. Renal trauma is found in 8% of penetrating abdominal wounds, with knives and gunshot wounds being the most prevalent.[9] In 80% of penetrating renal injuries, there will be associated intra-abdominal visceral injuries.[9]

Physical Examination

Physical findings consistent with potential renal trauma are flank contusions, lower rib fractures, lumbar vertebral fractures, upper abdominal tenderness, and any penetrating injury of the flank and upper abdomen.

The physical findings of ureteral injury are nonspecific and usually are the result of associated injuries. The diagnosis is based on suspicion. Ureteral injuries secondary to blunt trauma are rare.[10] A penetrating wound present along the course of the ureters should lead to a diagnostic workup to rule out ureteral injury.

Pelvic fractures may herald the presence of a bladder injury. Pelvic fractures with instability and crepitance on examination are associated with bladder rupture or urethral disruption in 20% of the cases.[11] Conversely, 90% of bladder ruptures have concomitant pelvic fractures and gross hematuria.[12] Gunshot and stab wounds to the lower abdomen may also result in injury to the bladder. The patient will typically present with lower abdominal pain and is unable to void.

Blood at the urethral meatus may be the only physical finding of urethral injury.[13] A high-riding prostate on rectal examination and scrotal hematoma may also indicate urethral trauma. All of these findings should be investigated via a retrograde urethrogram prior to the introduction of a Foley catheter to avoid further damage to an injured urethra.

Diagnostic Tests

Urinalysis

The initial test that should be obtained in the evaluation of the urinary system is a urine sample. This should be obtained as early in the patient's course as possible. Atraumatic catheterization of the bladder should be performed if not contraindicated by the presence of blood at the urethral meatus, scrotal hematoma, or high-riding or absent prostate on rectal examination. The first 30 cc should be discarded because it may be contaminated with blood from the passage of the catheter. The next aliquot should be tested for blood by dipstick and sent for complete urinalysis. A positive urine dipstick for blood correlates to 10 or more red blood cells/high power field (RBC/HPF) on urinalysis—adequate evidence of urinary system injury.[14]

Hematuria is the best indicator of urinary system injury. The presence of 5 RBC/HPF or positive urine dipstick should prompt the initiation of renal imaging. The degree of hematuria does not correspond to the severity of injury.[15] Of patients with renal artery thrombosis, 28% will present without hematuria.[16] Therefore, a good argument may be made for imaging the urinary system in all patients with a history of major deceleration accidents.[17]

Recently, there have been reports in the literature suggesting that *adult* patients who sustain blunt abdominal trauma may be selectively imaged.[18–20] Blunt trauma patients without shock (systolic blood pressure less than 90 mmHg) and with only microscopic hematuria may be observed without imaging. The determination of shock must begin in the field at the time of initial evaluation by the paramedics. All patients with shock and microscopic hematuria, and with gross hematuria regardless of blood pressure, should be imaged. These authors report safely avoiding imaging studies in 70% of adult patients with blunt trauma. However, patients with multiple associated abdominal injuries and suggestion of renal injury by examination or celiotomy should still be imaged. These criteria are *not* applicable to children, and patients with penetrating trauma. All patients with microscopic hematuria and penetrating trauma should undergo renal imaging.

It is the author's opinion that this selective course is fraught with some danger. As has already been stated, a quarter of the most severe renal injuries, pedicle injuries, will present without microscopic hematuria. Applying the selective criteria would result in the missed diagnosis of these injuries, and the needless loss of kidneys and increased incidence of complications due to these missed injuries. Logically, the safest course would be to obtain renal imaging based on microscopic hematuria (more than 5 RBC/HPF) and mechanism of injury.

With ureteral injuries, 90% will show microscopic hematuria, and 10% will show no hematuria.[21] Bladder injuries usually present with gross hematuria and microscopic hematuria will almost always be present. Again, the need for imaging even with microscopic hematuria, especially in penetrating trauma, is emphasized.

As previously pointed out, the single best indicator of urethral trauma is blood at the urethral meatus. Even the slightest amount of blood should prompt imaging of the urethra prior to the insertion of a catheter.

Intravenous Pyelography

Intravenous pyelography (IVP) represents the basic diagnostic test in the evaluation and staging of injuries to the urinary system. The test should be obtained in those trauma patients who present with microscopic hematuria (more than 5 RBC/HPF) or have significant mechanism of injury, as has been previously discussed, even in the absence of hematuria.

The most efficient method of performing the IVP is the "one shot" technique. This method may be used even in severely injured patients and should not add any time to the initial resuscitation and evaluation. In the more stable patient, a formal IVP may be obtained. After the placement of large bore resuscitation intravenous catheters, high-dose renal contrast medium, 2.0 cc/kg, should be infused with the initial resuscitation fluids as a bolus. A flat plate abdominal radiograph should be obtained approximately 10 minutes after the contrast has been delivered. This film will usually demonstrate bilateral nephrograms, the collecting systems, and contrast medium in the ureters.

Fine detail of the urinary system may not be obtained using this technique, but in the unstable patient valuable information will be gained prior to surgical exploration. The functional status of both renal units will be ascertained, and possible extravasation identified.

Delayed visualization may be indicative of a renal contusion or minor parenchymal laceration. Unilateral nonvisualization is indicative of a major renal injury, usually a renal pedicle injury. This finding mandates further imaging to delineate the injury, as will be discussed subsequently. Bilateral nonvisualization is rare and usually is found with bilateral renal artery thrombosis. These patients will demonstrate no urine output. Partial nonvisualization of a single renal unit usually indicates an injury in that segment of the kidney. Again, further studies will be necessary to delineate the injury. Extravasation may be noted and, in the stable patient, delayed films will be helpful to define the extent of the extravasation.

A criticism of IVP is the accuracy of the test in establishing a definitive diagnosis, only 50% in some series.[22] However, the use of high-dose contrast medium has improved the yield. In the unstable patient even the minimal information of bilateral renal function is important to the surgeon in planning intraoperative strategies. The addition of nephrotomography in the stable patient has proven to yield a diagnosis in 90% of patients.[23] This study delineates the renal outline and is particularly accurate in defining intrarenal hematomas and parenchymal lacerations.

Information on ureteral injuries may also be found on the IVP. An injured ureter may be demonstrated by delayed visualization, mild hydronephrosis, and extravasation of contrast.[24] When ureteral injury is suspected on IVP, retrograde ureterogram should be performed to define the injury accurately.

Bladder injuries are usually not well defined by IVP, although occasionally extravasation from a bladder rupture may be seen. In suspected bladder injury, IVP should not be utilized as the primary diagnostic modality. A cystogram should be performed to make the diagnosis.

Other Contrast Studies

Cystography.   A cystogram should be obtained in every trauma patient in whom there is evidence of severe intra-abdominal trauma with hematuria, or with a pelvic fracture and hematuria. After examination has cleared the urethra, or a retrograde urethrogram has demonstrated an intact urethra, a Foley catheter should be passed into the bladder. The bladder is gravity filled with 350 to 400 cc of 50% contrast media. Three films should be obtained to examine the bladder accurately. The initial film is made as an anteroposterior radiograph with the bladder filled. A second film is made with the bladder full and is taken as a cross-table lateral or an oblique radiograph to visualize the posterior bladder. A third film is made after the bladder is emptied via gravity drainage. Fifteen percent of bladder injuries will be extraperitoneal and not visualized except on the lateral/oblique or postemptying views.[25]

Retrograde Urethrography.   Urethrography should be obtained in every male trauma patient with evidence of blood at the meatus prior to attempting passage of a Foley catheter. If resistance is met when attempting gentle catheterization, a urethrogram should be obtained prior to proceeding with the attempt. The passage of a bladder catheter in the presence of a urethral injury may result in converting a partial disruption into a complete laceration, bacterial seeding of a pelvic hematoma, or increased fibrosis secondary to additional injury from the catheter. Additional injury, false passages, and strictures may result from the blind probing of a urethral injury with a catheter. The IVP may yield information that would lead to a urethrogram. If the bladder is found to be residing in an elevated position, a prompt urethrogram should be performed.

The technique of retrograde urethrography is simple, quick, requires no special equipment, and may be performed in the emergency department. An irrigating syringe is filled with 20 cc of undiluted contrast material, and the tip is inserted into the urethral meatus. The penis is stretched slightly to the side and the 20 cc of contrast medium is injected into the urethra. A lateral radiograph is obtained as the injection is completed. If a catheter has already been placed into the bladder and a urethral injury is subsequently suspected, a urethrogram should still be performed. This is accomplished by inserting a 5 F feeding tube or a 20 gauge intravenous catheter alongside the Foley catheter and injecting contrast as a lateral film is taken. The Foley catheter should not be removed, because it serves as a stent for the injured urethra.

The most common site of urethral disruption is at the prostatomembranous urethral junction. The prostatic urethra is severed from the membranous urethra at the level of the triangular ligament. Extravasation of contrast will be seen at the site of disruption; partial visualization of the prostatic urethra means that there is incomplete disruption. When complete disruption is present, there will be no passage of contrast medium into the prostatic urethra or bladder, and all contrast will be extravasated.

Arteriography.   Selective renal arteriography has been the traditional study to evaluate major renal and pelvic injuries. With the development of computed tomography (CT), arteriography has assumed a position lower on the diagnostic totem pole. This study should be obtained if CT is unavailable or not definitive in staging the renal injury. Partial or complete nonvisualization of a renal unit should lead to the suspicion of a major renal injury, and arteriography may be considered. Digital subtraction angiography appears to be as useful as conventional arteriography. Therapeutic arteriography with embolization may be considered when persistent arterial bleeding is present.

Computed Tomography

CT has completely revolutionized the diagnosis and treatment of urinary tract injuries. Accurate staging of injuries is now possible and more refined treatment schemes have been developed. CT defines the depth and extent of lacerations, is very sensitive for extravasation, depicts the size and extent of retroperitoneal hematomas, and detects many associated intra-abdominal injuries.[19] Renal artery injuries have also been accurately detected with CT,[26] but arteriography remains the diagnostic test of choice for pedicle injuries. For CT to be considered a reliable diagnostic tool in the trauma patient, it must be immediately available 24 hours a day, be a third generation or newer scanner, and an experienced trauma CT radiologist must be present for immediate interpretation. If these three criteria cannot be met, then other diagnostic tests must be relied on.

CT has several distinct advantages: (1) three-dimensional views; (2) noninvasiveness, in most patients; (3) excellent definition of parenchymal laceration; (4) sensitive detection of extravasation; (5) delineation of nonviable tissue; (6) definition of size and extent of perirenal hematoma; and (7) detection of associated injuries.[27] Because of the sensitivity of CT in detecting contrast extravasation, ureteral and bladder injuries may be detected, but CT should not be relied on to make these diagnoses. IVP remains the diagnostic test of choice for ureteral injuries, and cystography for bladder injuries.

Other Diagnostic Studies

Renal Scans.   Radioisotopic scans of the kidneys are helpful in detecting disrupted renal blood flow, but are otherwise unhelpful due to the lack of resolution in the scans. Availability in the emergency, trauma setting also limits the usefulness of these studies. **Renal Ultrasound.**   Ultrasonography has been espoused by the European literature,[28] but has been met with less than enthusiastic support in this country. The major deficiency with ultrasound is the inability to differentiate between hematoma, laceration, and urine.[27]

CLASSIFICATION AND OPERATIVE INDICATIONS

Using the algorithm in Figure 12–1, renal injuries may be accurately staged and the therapeutic approach planned, based on defined indications. Accurately classifying renal injuries also allows for the meaningful comparison of treatment protocols, whereby standards of therapy may be refined.

Minor renal injuries include contusions and superficial lacerations that extend only into the renal cortex (Fig. 12–2). Minor injuries account for 90% of all blunt renal injuries.[29]

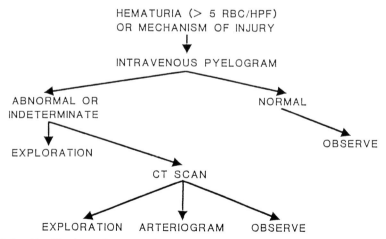

Figure 12–1.   Algorithm for renal trauma workup. RBC/HPF: red blood cells per high power field; CT: computed tomography.

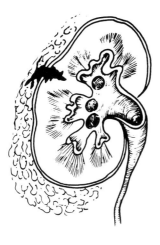
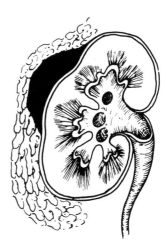

Figure 12–2. Minor class renal injuries.

These injuries are almost universally treated nonoperatively, and the kidney returns to normal on follow-up IVP.

Major injuries account for the remaining 10% of blunt renal trauma. Major injuries are comprised of: (1) lacerations that extend into the deep medulla without urine extravasation; (2) deep medullary lacerations that extend into the collecting system, resulting in urinary extravasation; and (3) renal pedicle injuries (Fig. 12–3). These injuries extend into the more highly vascularized regions of the kidney and are more likely to produce profound bleeding. Therefore these injuries are more likely to require operative intervention. However, the mere presence of a major injury does not, in itself, constitute an indication for mandatory exploration.[30] Approximately one half of major injuries may be treated nonoperatively.[31]

Specific operative indications have been developed and include: expanding or uncontained hematoma; pulsatile hematoma; major urinary extravasation; greater than 20% nonviable renal tissue; and renal pedicle injury.[32] Obviously, some of these indications are operative indications and others may be gained through nonoperative staging. Urinary extravasation is, in itself, not an absolute indication for renal exploration but is usually found in connection with other indications. Contrast extravasation beyond the renal capsule indicates significant damage to the collecting system. If nonoperative management is chosen for these patients, frequent (every 5 to 7 days) renal imaging should be performed to follow the progress of the urinoma. Any indication that the urinoma is infected should lead to prompt surgical drainage and repair of the defect.

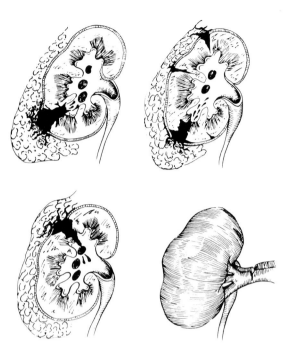

Figure 12–3. Major class renal injuries.

Most penetrating injuries will require operative exploration, unless noninvasive staging has yielded enough information to determine that nonoperative therapy will be sufficient.[33] Hemodynamically stable patients with penetrating flank injuries may undergo a staging workup consisting of IVP and CT scan. If poor visualization of the ipsilateral kidney is demonstrated on IVP and the CT shows a parenchymal laceration without involvement of the collecting system, then the patient may be safely followed nonoperatively. Using such a staging system and following the aforementioned surgical indications, McAninch and colleagues at San Francisco General Hospital have been able to follow 50% of patients with renal stab wounds and 15% with renal gunshot wounds.[4]

Any ureteral injury found on workup should undergo early exploration and repair to avoid late complications. The vast majority of ureteral injuries are secondary to penetrating trauma and have a high rate of associated injuries that also require surgical repair.

Intraperitoneal rupture of the bladder requires surgical exploration and repair with postoperative bladder drainage. Contained extraperitoneal bladder rupture may be followed nonoperatively and treated with bladder drainage.[34,35] A low-pressure cystogram is obtained after 14 days and repeated until no further extravasation is demonstrated. After the bladder has sealed, the urinary catheter may be removed.

Urethral injury does require immediate surgical attention. The preferred initial management is via suprapubic cystostomy for urinary diversion. This approach allows for the healing of associated injuries and fractures. In most patients with partial urethral disruption, the injury will heal with minimal stricture formation and formal repair is usually not necessary. The same is true for anterior urethral injuries. Complete prostato-membranous disruption may be repaired after a delay of 3 to 4 months. It is important that urologic consultation be obtained early when a urethral injury is identified.

OPERATIVE MANAGEMENT

Renal Injuries

As previously discussed in Chapter 5, the appropriate incision to make is a generous midline transabdominal one. In renal trauma the retroperitoneum is often distorted by the presence of a massive retroperitoneal hematoma. It is important to look carefully for anatomic landmarks that may not be in their accustomed locations.

When the decision is made, using the previously discussed indications, to perform renal exploration, it is important that renal vascular control be obtained prior to entering the perinephric hematoma. This is most easily and safely accomplished by exposing the aorta and inferior vena cava through the root of the small bowel mesentery (Fig. 12–4). The inferior mesenteric vein is a major landmark that must be identified in order to place properly the incision to open the retroperitoneum. This incision is made just medial to the inferior mesenteric vein and over the aorta. The incision extends up to the ligament of Treitz. Often the aorta will be involved in the hematoma, and by approaching the great vessels medial to the inferior mesenteric vein, the hematoma may be safely entered and the aorta identified. The only branch of the aorta at this level is the inferior mesenteric artery, and this may be easily avoided. The dissection is carried out on the anterior surface of the aorta until the left renal vein is found passing over the aorta. This is an important landmark because it marks the takeoff of the right and left renal arteries from the aorta. The paired arteries arise just superior to the left renal vein and from the lateral surfaces of the aorta. The vessels are dissected out and vessel loops passed around them. The right renal vein requires further dissection laterally to the inferior vena cava where it joins the vena cava on its right

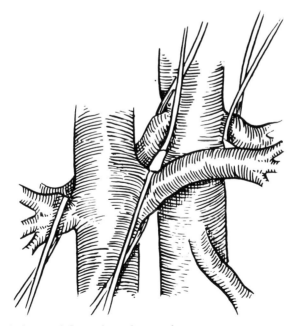

Figure 12–4. Surgical approach for renal vascular control.

lateral surface, opposite the left renal vein. All four major renal vessels can be easily isolated through this single incision.

The kidneys themselves are exposed by incising the peritoneal reflection lateral to the colon and rotating the colon medially to expose the perinephric hematoma. The kidney is bluntly dissected out of the hematoma to expose the kidney completely. If vascular control has been appropriately obtained prior to this point, then this dissection can be accomplished without major blood loss. If vascular occlusion is required to prevent major blood loss, then the warm ischemic time should be kept to less than 30 minutes. If longer ischemic times are anticipated, then the kidney should be cooled in its fossa with slush ice. By utilizing this technique for vascular control followed by renal exposure, the nephrectomy rate has been significantly lowered.[32]

Large intrarenal hematomas contained in lacerations should be removed and the injury carefully examined. Nonviable tissue must be debrided back to healthy, bleeding parenchyma. Hemostasis should be attained using suture ligature of individual arteries and veins. Fine chromic suture on a taper needle is most appropriate. Chromic passes through the tissue with less of a cutting tendency than braided synthetic sutures. Silk and other permanent sutures should never be used, for they act as niduses for stone formation and have a higher rate of secondary infection. If the collecting system has been violated, it must be closed in a watertight fashion. Again, it must be emphasized that chromic is the best suture for closing the collecting system for the reasons already cited.

Upper and lower pole injuries may require partial nephrectomy. After the edges are debrided, suture ligature is used for hemostasis and the collecting system is securely closed. Through-and-through mattress sutures to compress the wound edges should be avoided, for they cause ischemia and further tissue loss. Continued oozing from the raw edge can usually be controlled with manual compression and application of one of the absorbable microfibrillar collagen products.

The raw surfaces left after debridement of lacerations and partial nephrectomies need to be covered. Ideally, the renal capsule should be reapproximated, but this is often impossible when the capsule has been severely damaged in the injury. In this case the omentum makes an acceptable patch. A pedicle of omentum may be brought through the mesocolon and stitched to the site of injury.

Drainage of the retroperitoneum after renal repair is not mandatory and may lead to secondary infection of the hematoma. Drainage to prevent hematoma formation is fruitless. Drains are only left if the security of the closure of the collecting system is in doubt. This closure may be tested by occlusion of the proximal ureter and gentle injection of methylene blue through the ureter to fill the renal pelvis and calyces. Areas where the methylene blue leaks may be closed with additional interrupted sutures.

Renal artery injuries must be immediately repaired. If surgical intervention is delayed longer than 4 hours, the salvage rate is very low. The injured segment of the renal artery is removed and an interposition graft is placed. Saphenous vein and hypogastric artery are suitable graft materials. Autotransplantation has also been used with success.[36] Small infarctions of less than 15 to 20% may be safely left without fear of subsequent adverse sequelae. Larger infarctions must be debrided using the same techniques as discussed before. Repair of segmental renal arteries or accessory arteries is generally time consuming and not rewarding. They are best treated with ligation and removal of any subsequent nonviable tissue.

Lacerations of the main renal vein should be closed with fine vascular sutures.

Segmental veins may be safely ligated because the intrarenal collateral circulation is excellent.

Using these techniques for renal repair, the San Francisco group has had a very high rate of renal salvage.[32] They were able to reconstruct 82% of the kidneys operated on. For blunt trauma, the repair rate was 100% (14 of 14 patients), and for penetrating trauma, the rate was 72% (18 of 25 patients). No longer should nephrectomy be the mandatory outcome in explorations for major renal injuries.

Ureteral Injuries

The vast majority of patients with an injury to the ureter have had penetrating trauma and will require abdominal exploration to repair associated injuries. It is usually most expedient to repair the other intra-abdominal injuries first, prior to proceeding with exploration and repair of the ureteral injury. The ipsilateral colon is mobilized medially to expose the course of the involved ureter. The area of injury must be carefully inspected to ascertain the amount of debridement that will be required to remove all devitalized tissue. Care should be taken to mobilize only as much ureter as is absolutely necessary to make a complete inspection in order to avoid devascularization of the remaining ureter.

The principles of repair for ureteral injuries are very similar to the general principles that should be adhered to in the formation of any anastomosis.[37] It is mandatory that the injury be adequately debrided; the anastomosis should be tension-free, spatulated, and watertight; ureteral stents should be placed; and the retroperitoneum in the region of the anastomosis should be adequately drained (Fig. 12–5). Very small lacerations with good wound edges may be primarily closed with interrupted fine chromic sutures. Chromic suture is used in ureteral repairs for the same reasons as already cited in the section on repair of renal injuries.

Injuries that are located in the lower third of the ureter are best managed by reimplantation into the bladder through a submucosal tunnel. This technique has the advantage of reducing or eliminating reflux. Should it appear that the reimplantation will be under undue tension, then a bladder hitch should be performed. The bladder on the ipsilateral side is pulled up and sutured to the fascia of the psoas muscle to relieve the tension. Primary reanastomosis may also be possible in the distal third. A spatulated anastomosis is performed in order to avoid stricture formation at the repair site.

When injuries involve the mid or upper thirds of the ureter, the repair of choice is primary ureteroureterostomy. The devitalized portion of the ureter is debrided and the proximal and distal segments are dissected free for a distance adequate to ensure a tension-free anastomosis. A double "J" internal silicone catheter stent should be placed through the injury site, proximal to the renal pelvis and distal into the bladder, prior to the performance of the anastomosis. Fine interrupted chromic sutures are used to make the spatulated anastomosis. The internal catheter stent may be left in place for several weeks and removed via simple cystoscopy. These catheter stents aid in maintaining alignment of the repair, assures patency of the ureter through the healing process, and prevents urinary extravasation through the repair site.

Occasionally, injuries will be encountered where a long segment of the ureter has been lost and primary repair will be impossible. This type of injury may require that a transureteroureterostomy be performed. If the patient's condition does not allow for the

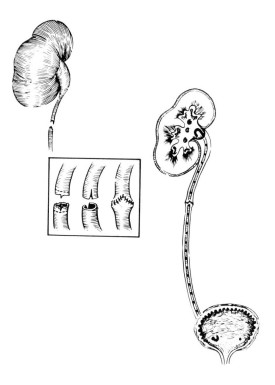

Figure 12–5. Essentials of ureteral repair.

performance of the repair at the time of initial exploration, a diverting nephrostomy may be done and the repair performed in 2 to 3 months. It is important to follow some basic principles when performing this type of repair. The contralateral ureter should be exposed with as little manipulation as possible to preserve its blood supply. A longitudinal 2.0 cm ureterotomy is made and the ipsilateral ureter anastomosed with fine interrupted chromic sutures.

If none of the methods just discussed is feasible, the ureter may be replaced with an ileal conduit; autotransplantation is another acceptable alternative.

Drainage of the retroperitoneum should be performed when ureteral repair has been performed. Closed system drain should be employed to minimize the chances for secondary infection along the drain tract, and the drains should be removed as early as possible for the same reason.

Bladder Injuries

Certain injuries to the bladder may be treated nonoperatively as long as certain criteria are met.[34,35] The rupture must be confined to the retroperitoneal space, with no evidence of extravasation into the free peritoneal cavity. Secondly, the urine must be sterile at the time of the injury. If both of these conditions are met, then the treatment of choice is bladder drainage via urethral catheter. After 2 weeks, a low-pressure cystogram is performed and drainage is maintained if there is evidence of continued extravasation. Cystography is repeated weekly until the bladder has healed. The risks of this approach are discontinuing drainage prior to healing of the bladder and secondary infection of the pelvic hematoma via the bladder. The first complication is avoided by monitoring healing via cystography, as explained before, and the second is minimized by careful catheter care.

Intraperitoneal ruptures of the bladder must be repaired during surgical exploration. Isolated bladder ruptures do occur, but a thorough exploration of the abdomen should always be carried out to rule out associated injuries. Almost all intraperitoneal bladder injuries are present on the dome of the bladder and are easily visualized from the standard, midline incision. The operative repair of these injuries is usually straightforward and may be accomplished with minimal complications.[12] If the defect is small, it should be enlarged to permit complete examination of the bladder for other injuries. Extraperitoneal lacerations are repaired from within using a single-layer absorbable interrupted suture. If the laceration extends into the bladder neck, the repair must be meticulously performed in order to reconstruct the sphincter mechanism and avoid urinary incontinence. The ureteral orifices must be carefully examined for any potential injuries. If doubt exists as to the patency of the ureteral orifices, the patient may be given 5.0 cc of indigo carmine intravenously and the ureters observed for the dye, which should appear within 10 minutes. Catheters may also be placed into the ureters and checked for the finding of clear urine from above.

The intraperitoneal bladder lacerations may be closed in two layers. The first incorporates the mucosa and bladder muscle, and the second the bladder muscle and peritoneum. Once the repair is complete a suprapubic cystostomy tube is placed in the anterior extraperitoneal position. The anterior surface of the bladder is exposed via dissection in the space of Retzius and a purse-string suture is placed through which the catheter is inserted. The catheter is brought out through a separate stab wound lateral to the midline incision and secured to the skin. Retropubic drains are unnecessary and should be avoided due to the risk of secondary infection along the drain tract.

Cystostomy drainage is maintained for 1 to 2 weeks to clear the gross hematuria and allow the bladder time to seal. This catheter may be left in place for extended periods of time if associated injuries are going to keep the patient in bed.

Urethral Injuries

The initial management of urethral injuries is urinary diversion via catheter drainage of the bladder. This is usually accomplished with a suprapubic cystostomy. A small, low, midline incision is made and the anterior wall of the bladder is exposed. The anterior bladder is opened and the interior surface of the bladder inspected for injuries. These are repaired as already described if they are encountered. The anterior wall is closed in two layers around a 26 F catheter. No drains are used in order to avoid secondary contamination of the pelvic hematoma. An alternative method is the use of percutaneous suprapubic catheters, but these have two disadvantages. First, they are small and make prolonged drainage difficult, and, second, they do not allow for inspection of the bladder for associated injuries.

Cystostomy drainage is continued for at least 3 months, or until all associated injuries are healed and the patient is in condition to undergo the formal stricture repair. Not all patients, those with incomplete posterior or anterior urethral injuries, will require formal repair. A voiding cystogram performed via the cystostomy tube will be invaluable in determining those patients who require repair. Many types of urethral repairs and reconstructions are available. These should be performed by an experienced urologist familiar with the varied techniques, so that the repair may be tailored to the needs of the particular injury. Since these injuries do not require immediate repair, and may wait until the patient is sent to an experienced urologist, these techniques will not be addressed in this text.

COMPLICATIONS

Renal Injuries

The outcome of repair of renal injuries should be good. It may be expected that 88% of kidneys operated on for major blunt or penetrating injuries may be salvaged.[38] Major renal pedicle injuries appear to be an exception to this bright outlook. The literature has established that few kidneys with such injuries may be salvaged.

Persistent urinary drainage from the closed system drains placed at surgery may represent urine or peritoneal fluid. The creatinine content of such drainage should be determined to make the differentiation. If drainage persists for greater than 1 week, an IVP should be obtained to determine adequacy of the repair and rule out distal obstruction. Poor closure technique and distal obstruction may account for the drainage. Continuing closed system drainage and removing any distal obstruction will normally result in closure of the leak.

Hypertension is an uncommon, but real, complication of renal injuries and may occur even in patients with contusions and other minor injuries. This occurs in less than 5% of patients. The onset may be delayed by 10 to 15 years, but usually is manifested within 12 to 18 months. Patients should be followed with occasional blood pressure checks to monitor for this complication.

Ureteral Injuries

Fistula formation is rare following ureteral repair but may occur if distal obstruction or stricture develops. Either condition requires correction before the fistula may be expected to close. Persistent urinary drainage without demonstrable stricture or obstruction may be managed by inserting a catheter stent for diversion, and the fistula will then spontaneously close. Rarely do urinary fistulas require operative intervention.

Hydronephrosis from stricture formation at the site of repair may occur. This may develop slowly over several months. Patients should be followed with IVP at 6 weeks and 3 months after stent removal to follow ureteral healing.

If the diagnosis of ureteral injury is delayed, the patient will probably develop a urinoma secondary to the retroperitoneal urinary extravasation. This complication should be suspected in the patient with a penetrating flank injury who has a persistent ileus, low-grade fever, and flank pain. This requires exploration, ureteral repair, and closed system drainage of the retroperitoneum at the site of the injury.

Urinary tract infections in these patients may be devastating. Infections may result in abscess formation, retroperitoneal scarring, and pyelonephritis. Periodic urine cultures should be obtained and, if positive, aggressive antibiotic therapy instituted.

Bladder Injuries

Complications of bladder injuries are rare due to the bladder's excellent blood supply and potential for recovery. Any aberrations in micturition, such as frequency or urgency, are usually self-limiting. Cystitis may be easily treated with antibiotics. Fistulas at the suprapubic catheter site are rare and usually herald the presence of a urethral obstruction, secondary to a missed urethral injury. The mortality rate with bladder injuries is reported to be high (22%), but this represents the severity of the associated injuries normally present.[12]

Urethral Injuries

The most severe complications of urethral injuries are stricture, impotence, and incontinence. By delaying the formal repair for several months through the use of suprapubic cystostomy, the impotence rate has been lowered to 10 to 20%.[4] Stricture formation only occurs in less than 10% of patients when careful repair by an experienced urologist has been performed. Short strictures may be treated with direct vision urethrotomy. Incontinence was as high as 33% but has now been lowered to less than 5% with good technique.[4] Stricture formation is the most common complication of anterior urethral injuries, with impotence and incontinence only rarely occurring.

SUMMARY

Injuries to the genitourinary system often occur in the trauma patient. The majority of these injuries are minor and will not require operative intervention. However, major renal injuries, ureteral lacerations, bladder ruptures, and urethral disruptions may have devastating complications if not found and treated early. Therefore aggressive diagnostic workup is mandatory. Microscopic hematuria must be pursued by obtaining an IVP. If renal injury is suspected from the IVP, careful staging should be done via CT. Arteriography is performed if vascular injury is suspected. Ureteral injuries will usually be found on IVP. Cystography may be necessary to demonstrate bladder rupture. Retrograde urethrography is mandatory if there is blood at the urethral meatus, scrotal hematoma, or high-riding prostate on rectal examination to rule out urethral injury.

Surgical repair of urinary tract injuries may be carried out with the expectation of excellent results and acceptable complication rates. Nephrectomy should not be the anticipated outcome of major renal injuries requiring exploration after careful staging. Up to 90% of these kidneys should be salvaged.

REFERENCES

1. Mendez R: Renal trauma. *J Urol* 1977;118:698–703.
2. McAninch JW: Injuries to the urinary system. In Blaisdell WF, Trunkey DD (eds): *Trauma Management, vol. I: Abdominal Trauma*. New York: Thieme-Stratton, 1982, p 199.
3. Peters PC, Bright TC III: Blunt renal injuries. *Urol Clin North Am* 1977;4:17.
4. McAninch JW: Genitourinary trauma. In Mattox KL, Moore EE, Feliciano DV (eds): *Trauma*. Norwalk, CT: Appleton and Lange, 1988, pp 537–552.

5. Chopart M: Traité des Malades des Voies Urinaires. Paris, France, Croullebois, 1792, p 88.
6. Evans E, Fowler HA: Puncture wounds of the bladder. *Ann Surg* 1905;42:215.
7. Hinman F: *Principles and Practice of Urology*. Philadelphia: WB Saunders, 1936, p 398.
8. Paré A: *The Apologie and Treatise of Ambroise Paré*. Birmingham, AL: Classics of Surgery Library, 1984, pp 55–59.
9. Carlton CE Jr, Scott R Jr, Goldman M: The management of penetrating injuries of the kidney. *J Trauma* 1968;8:1071–1083.
10. Heath AD, May A: Bilateral avulsion of the upper ureter. *Br J Urol* 1975;47:386.
11. Palmer JK, Benson GS, Corriere JN Jr: Diagnosis and initial management of urological injuries associated with 200 consecutive pelvic fractures. *J Urol* 1983;130:712–714.
12. Carroll PR, McAninch JW: Bladder trauma: Mechanisms of injury and a unified method of diagnosis and repair. *J Urol* 1984;132:254–257.
13. McAninch JW: Traumatic injuries to the urethra. *J Trauma* 1981;21:291–297.
14. Chandhoke PS, McAninch JW: Detection and significance of microscopic hematuria in patients with blunt renal trauma. *J Urol* 1988;140:16–18.
15. Bright TC, White K, Peters PC: Significance of hematuria after trauma. *J Urol* 1978;120:455–456.
16. Stables DP, Fouche RF, de Villiers Van Niekerk JP, et al: Traumatic renal artery occlusion: 21 cases. *J Urol* 1976;115:229.
17. Cass AS, Burrick M, Luxenberg M, et al: Renal pedicle injuries in patients with multiple injuries. *J Trauma* 1985;25:892–896.
18. Cass AS: Immediate radiologic and surgical management of renal injuries. *J Trauma* 1982;22:361–363.
19. McAninch JW, Federle MP: Evaluation of renal injuries with computerized tomography. *J Urol* 1982;128:456–460.
20. Herschorn S, Radom SB, Shoskes DA, et al: Evaluation and treatment of blunt renal trauma. *J Urol* 1991;146:274–277.
21. Carlton CE Jr, Scott R Jr, Guthrie AG: The initial management of ureteral injuries: A report of 78 cases. *J Urol* 1971;105:335–340.
22. Lang EK: Arteriography in the assessment of renal trauma. The impact of arteriographic diagnosis on preservation of renal function and parenchyma. *J Trauma* 1975;15:553–566.
23. Mahoney SA, Persky L: Intravenous drip nephrotomography as an adjunct in the evaluation of renal injury. *J Urol* 1968;99:513–516.
24. Peterson NE, Pitts JC III: Penetrating injuries of the ureter. *J Urol* 1981;126:587–590.
25. Carroll PR, McAninch JW: Major bladder trauma: The accuracy of cystography. *J Urol* 1983;130:887–888.
26. Steinberg DL, Jeffrey RF, Federle MP, et al: The computerized tomography appearance of renal pedicle injury. *J Urol* 1984;132:1163–1164.
27. McAninch JW: Renal injuries. In Blaisdell FW, Trunkey DD, McAninch JW (eds): *Trauma Management, vol. II: Urogenital Trauma*. New York: Thieme-Stratton, 1985, pp 33–34.
28. Schmoller H, Kunit G, Frick J: Sonography in blunt renal trauma. *Eur Urol* 1981;7:11–15.
29. Nicolaisen GS, McAninch JW, Marshall G, et al: Renal trauma: Re-evaluation of indications for radiographic assessment. *J Urol* 1985;133:183–187.
30. Meretyk S, Shapiro A, Lebensart PD: Conservative treatment in severe renal trauma. *Urology* 1991;37:251–252.
31. Peterson NE: Intermediate-degree blunt renal trauma. *J Trauma* 1977;17:425–435.
32. McAninch JW, Carroll PR: Renal trauma: Kidney preservation through improved vascular control—A refined approach. *J Trauma* 1982;22:285–290.
33. Carroll PR, McAninch JW: Operative indications in penetrating renal trauma. *J Trauma* 1985;25:587–593.
34. Hayes EE, Sandler CM, Corriere JN Jr: Management of the ruptured bladder secondary to blunt abdominal trauma. *J Urol* 1983;129:946–948.
35. Cass AS, Johnson CF, Kahn AU, et al: Nonoperative management of the bladder rupture from external trauma. *Urology* 1983;22:27–29.
36. Fay R, Brosman S, Lindstrom R, et al: Renal artery thrombosis: A successful revascularization by autotransplantation. *J Urol* 1974;111:572–577.
37. Carlton CE Jr, Guthrie AG, Scott R Jr: Surgical correction of ureteral injury. *J Trauma* 1969;9:457–464.
38. Carroll PR, Klosterman PW, McAninch JW: Surgical management of renal trauma: Analysis of risk factors, technique, and outcome. *J Trauma* 1988;28:1071–1077.

13

Pelvic Fractures

MICHAEL J. BOSSE, M.D., F.A.C.S.
CHARLES M. REINERT, M.D.

The recognition of the unstable pelvic fracture as a harbinger of a potentially lethal injury complex has led to the development of aggressive preemptive treatment protocols for patients with this injury. Hemorrhage remains the leading cause of death in pelvic fractures, with the overall mortality rate greater than 15%. McMurtry et al[1] reported that the combination of a pelvic fracture and an intracranial mass lesion requiring neurosurgical intervention had an associated mortality of 50%; a pelvic fracture associated with a hemorrhagic intra-abdominal injury requiring celiotomy had a mortality rate of 52%; and the combination of pelvic fracture, an intracranial mass lesion, and an intra-abdominal injury had a mortality rate exceeding 90%. The awareness of the hemorrhagic complications of pelvic fracture[2–8] and of associated skeletal, intracranial, respiratory, urogenital, and abdominal injuries (Table 13–1) has hastened the efforts to make the diagnosis of a pelvic fracture in the blunt trauma patient.

Significant forces are required to disrupt the pelvic ring. The recent MIEMSS (Maryland Institute for Emergency Medical Services Systems) experience[9] reported the trauma etiology as: motor vehicle accident: 57%; motorcycle accident: 8.9%; falls: 9.6%; pedestrian: 12.5%; and crush: 3.5%. Motor vehicle crashes were the common cause of lateral compression injuries, while anterior compression injuries were commonly caused by crush. A zone of injury is defined as the pelvic fractures or dislocations, and the impact forces dissipated into the soft tissues.

Injury to pelvic viscera results from the forces of impact, or secondarily, from displacement of sharp fracture fragments, or cephalad migration of the entire hemipelvis. Dalal et al,[9] among others,[10–12] has demonstrated the correlation between specific fracture patterns and the patient's clinical presentation and course. The direction and magnitude of the injury forces are delineated on the initial radiographs and are primary determinants of the pattern and severity of visceral injuries. "Acting together, the sequelae of those injuries set the physiologic severity, mandate the volume replacement needs and define the significant complications which ultimately lead to survival or death."[9] The high energy, unstable fractures are at greatest risk for hemorrhage and associated injuries.

Successful management of the pelvic fracture patient requires prompt recognition of the fracture, rapid identification of the patient at risk for severe hemorrhage, and prompt treatment. A coordinated effort must exist to manage multispecialty-associated injuries. Recognition of the contribution that the orthopedic surgeon can make to both the resuscita-

Table 13–1   Associated Injuries

SERIES	NO. PT	MOR-TALITY (%)	OPEN (%)	SKEL-ETAL (%)	HEAD (%)	RESPI-RATORY (%)	UROL-OGY (%)	ABDOM-INAL (%)	CARDIO-VASCULAR (%)
Trunkey et al,[10] 1974	173	9.2	—	86	13	34	7.5	18	—
Rothenberger et al,[41] 1978	604	12	4	—	—	—	11	14	1
McMurtry et al,[1] 1980	79	19	—	85	46	62	12	29	6
Naam et al,[8] 1983	102	17	13	61	43	32	11	25	7

tion effort and postresuscitative care of the pelvic fracture patient ranks as one of the most significant advances of the past decade in the management of these patients. Acute stabilization of the pelvis by external fixation has significantly decreased hemorrhagic mortality rates and requirements for blood products.[13–15] Further reduction in long-term mortality is realized by rapid mobilization of the patient.[16–18]

PATIENT EVALUATION

Clinical

A pelvic fracture must be suspected in every trauma patient with blunt trauma, crush, or fall as the mechanism of injury. The Advanced Trauma Life Support (ATLS) protocol[19] emphasizes the required physical examination and resuscitation principles. Physical findings specific for pelvic injuries include: genital ecchymosis and swelling; rectal, vaginal, or urethral bleeding; flank or sacral pain, ecchymosis or swelling; open wounds over the flank or in the perineum; and abnormal neurologic findings in the lower extremities. Palpation over the pubic rami, the symphysis, or the sacroiliac (SI) joint will elicit pain in the conscious patient. The displaced fracture fragments or the separated symphysis are often palpable. Instability of the hemipelvis can be demonstrated by provocative maneuvers: anterior pressure over the anterior iliac spines opens the pelvis and lateral pressure over the iliac wings closes the pelvis. Demonstrated motion signifies pelvic instability.

Pelvic fractures are associated with a 12% incidence of urogenital injuries and a 25% incidence of intra-abdominal injury. Prior to placing a urinary catheter, the urethral meatus, rectum, and vagina must be examined to exclude occult injury. In the male patient, meatal blood or a boggy, high-riding prostate are significant findings, indicative of a probable membranous urethral tear.[19] A retrograde urethrogram should be performed prior to placement of a transurethral urinary catheter. Blood in the rectum or the vagina is often caused by an open pelvic fracture, with fragments lacerating the rectal or vaginal tissues.

A peritoneal lavage will be required in most patients, because of associated hemodynamic instability or simply because of the mechanism of injury. Per the ATLS protocol, drainage of the bladder should be obtained prior to lavage. In patients with pelvic fractures, the lavage should be performed supraumbilical, with the catheter directed into the pelvis.[14,20]

Unstable pelvic fractures or fractures that involve the sacral ala or foramina risk injury to the lumbosacral plexus. A 20% incidence of lumbosacral plexus injury was reported by Winquist and Mayo[21] in a series of unstable pelvic fracture patients. Documentation of function of the sciatic, pudendal, and gluteal nerves is required.

Radiographic

Recognized by the American College of Surgeons' Committee on Trauma as an essential initial diagnostic radiograph, the anteroposterior (AP) pelvic film (Fig. 13–1) is obtained by most large trauma centers,[9,11,12,22] because a positive finding has both immediate prognostic and therapeutic implications.[10,22] Young and Burgess[11] found that the diagnosis and correct classification of the pelvic fracture could be made on review of the initial AP film in 90% of their cases.

Recognition of fracture or ligamentous instability on the initial AP radiograph requires augmentation views to confirm the fracture, the fracture mechanism, classification, and degree of posterior pelvic ring stability. In the secondary survey phase of the ATLS protocol, inlet (Fig. 13–2) and outlet (Fig. 13–3) views of the pelvis should be obtained. The inlet view helps to determine the amount of distraction of the pelvic ring, displacement of the fracture fragments, detect the horizontal fracture line at the pubic ramus seen in lateral compression injuries, and helps to identify an anterior crush component of the sacral ala. The pelvic outlet film helps to determine the posterior and superior displacement of the iliac wing in reference to the sacrum. Radiographs of the lumbosacral spine should also be obtained because of the high incidence of associated fractures.

Pelvic fractures are classified orthopedically as stable or unstable. Stability is based on the integrity of the posterior pelvic ring. Division of the pubic symphysis allows the pelvic ring to open only 2.5 cm if the posterior structures are intact. Additional external rotation forces, applied to the hemipelvis, disrupts the sacrospinous and the sacrotuberous ligaments, allowing the pelvis to open until the posterior superior iliac space abuts the sacrum.[23] Vertical displacement of the hemipelvis, however, cannot occur until the sacrotuberous ligament and the posterior sacroiliac ligamentous complex are disrupted (Fig. 13–4). Radiographic signs of pelvic instability include:

1. Displacement of the posterior sacroiliac complex more than 5 mm
2. Presence of posterior fracture gap, rather than impaction
3. Presence of avulsion fractures of the transverse process of the fifth lumbar vertebra, or the sacral or ischial end of the sacrospinous ligament

The integrity of the posterior pelvic ring determines the stability of the pelvic fracture. A computed tomographic (CT) scan (Fig. 13–5) is the best method to assess the degree of damage or displacement of the posterior ring.[24] Multiple trauma patients with pelvic fractures having CT scans to assess other injuries should not miss the opportunity to have at least 2 cuts obtained at the levels of the first sacral body. In patients in whom the stability of the pelvis is uncertain, push-pull radiographs can demonstrate the absence of stability

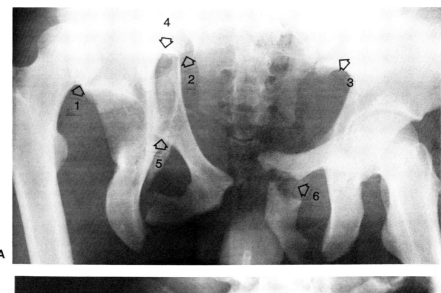

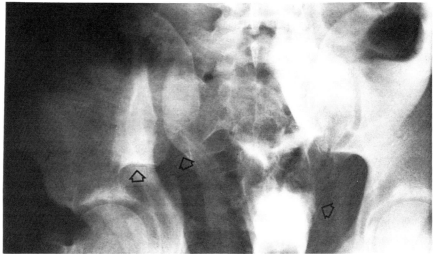

Figure 13–1. **A:** Even this poor quality admission pelvic radiograph provides significant information: 1: the hip is dislocated; 2, 3: bilateral widening of the sacroiliac joints; 4: suggestion of a posterior iliac wing fracture; 5: anterior column acetabular fracture; and 6: superior and inferior pubic ramus fractures. **B:** The hip was emergently reduced and a cystogram was obtained because of hematuria. This repeat anteroposterior radiograph shows a bladder disruption, a significantly displaced iliac wing fracture involving the sciatic notch, and unstable joints.

of the posterior sacroiliac complex.[25] McMurtry et al[1] identified a significant correlation between posterior pelvic disruption and patient mortality.

The following modification of Pennal et al's[26] classification of pelvic fractures, based on pattern and mechanism of injury, is most useful.

1. *Anteroposterior Compression.* The AP compression injury results from direct or indirect compression forces applied to the anterior or the posterior aspect of the pelvic ring.

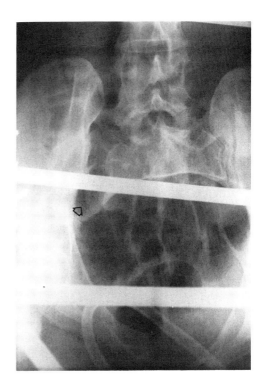

Figure 13–2. The inlet pelvic projection is obtained by directing the x-ray beam cephalad-caudad at an angle of 40° to the x-ray plate, with the beam centered at midpelvis. This inlet view obtained after "reduction" and application of an anterior external fixator demonstrates gross instability of the right hemipelvis with evidence of significant posterior translation at both the sacroiliac joint (arrow) and pubic symphysis.

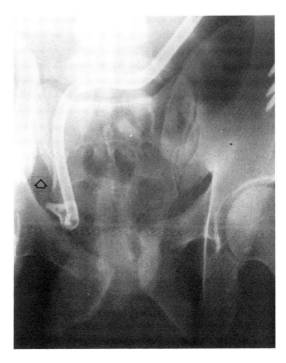

Figure 13–3. The pelvic outlet projection is obtained by directing the x-ray beam from caudad-cephalad at an angle of 40° to the x-ray plate with the beam centered on the symphysis. This projection gives an excellent view of the sacrum, sacroiliac joint, and symphysis. Note the grossly widened, dislocated right SI joint and proximal migration of the hemipelvis.

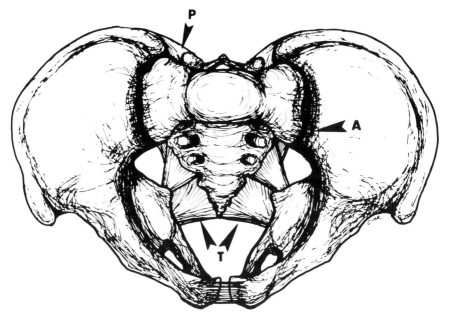

Figure 13–4.   Stability of the pelvic ring is maintained by integrity of the osseous structures, by the symphysis pubis, the posterior sacroiliac ligaments (P), the anterior sacroiliac ligaments (A), and the sacrotuberous and sacrospinous ligaments (T). (Reprinted with permission from Young and Burgess.[11])

The anterior forces can be transmitted through the femoral shaft to the acetabulum and iliac wings. Tile[23] prefers to call the forces external rotation forces, tending to disrupt the anterior pelvis and "open book" the pelvic ring. The AP compression injuries have been classified into three groups:[11,27]

> Type I. Minor diastasis of the symphysis and/or vertical fractures of the pubic rami.
>
> Type II. The pubic symphysis is open more than 2.5 cm. The pelvis "opens" because of injury to the anterior sacroiliac, sacrospinous, and sacrotuberus ligaments.
>
> Type III. There is a complete disruption of the sacroiliac joint and the pubic symphysis is widely separated. The hemipelvis is grossly unstable and can migrate laterally, posteriorly, or superiorly (Fig. 13–6).

2.   *Lateral Compression.* The lateral compression injury results from a direct impaction force on the iliac wing or from forces transmitted through the femur from a lateral impact over the greater trochanter. Young et al[28] have subclassified these injuries into three categories.

> Type I. The force is delivered to the lateral posterior aspect of the pelvic ring. All patients have horizontal pubic ramus fractures, best visualized on the pelvic inlet view. The posterior ligaments remain intact, and the fracture is usually stable.

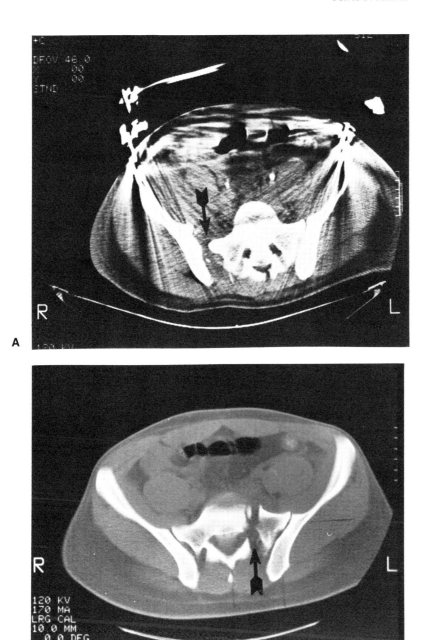

Figure 13–5.   **A:** The CT scan shows a complete disruption of the soft tissue of the posterior right hemipelvis, with widening and anterior dislocation of the SI joint (arrow). **B:** This patient's CT demonstrates an unstable sacral fracture pattern, with widening of the fracture site exceeding 10 mm (arrow).

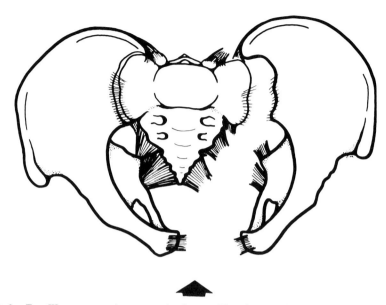

Figure 13–6. Type III: anteroposterior compression fracture. There is a complete disruption of the SI joint and symphysis pubis, with disruption of all major ligamentous support. The hemipelvis is grossly unstable and can migrate laterally, superiorly, and posteriorly. The usual injury vector is depicted by the arrow. (Reprinted with permission from Young and Burgess.[11])

Type II. The force is applied more anterior on the lateral pelvis, medially displacing the ipsilateral anterior hemipelvis. The posterior hemipelvis pivots around the sacral ala. An anterior crush fracture of the sacrum may occur. The soft tissue can disrupt posteriorly under the tensile strain, or the internal rotation force can cause a fracture through the iliac wing. This injury pattern is unstable.

Type III. Most severe form of a lateral compression injury resulting in a bilateral disruption of the pelvic ring. The force is applied anterolateral, causing an internal rotation of the anterior hemipelvis. The force continues through to the contralateral pelvis, causing an external rotation force-AP compression injury to the opposite hemipelvis (Fig. 13–7).

3. *Vertical Shear.* Also termed the "Malgaigne fracture," the vertical shear injury results from a severe vertical disruption force to the hemipelvis, such as the force a jumper would sustain. The posterior elements are disrupted by either sacral or iliac wing fractures or by ligamentous disruption of the sacroiliac joint. The pelvis is unstable (Fig. 13–8).
4. *Complex/Combined Patterns.* Pelvic injuries resulting from a mixed force vector application.
5. *Associated Fractures.* Isolated iliac wing fractures, pubic rami fractures, and acetabular fractures are not without complications. They have potential for visceral and vascular injury[29,30] and often require open reduction and internal fixation.

In a review of 350 pelvic fractures, Young and Burgess[11] found that 49% of their patients had lateral compression injuries, 21% had anterior compression injuries, 6% had

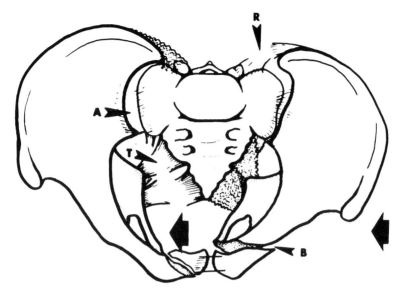

Figure 13–7. Type III: lateral compression fracture. The force is applied anteriorly on the iliac wing (arrow) causing an internal rotation of the anterior hemipelvis. The ipsilateral hemipelvis hinges on the sacral ala, causing a compression fracture there and disrupting the posterior ligament complex (R). The force continues through to the contralateral pelvis, causing it to externally rotate, and producing an anteroposterior compression-like injury there, with disruption of the sacrotuberous—sacrospinous ligament complex (T) and of the anterior sacroiliac ligaments (A). The "horizontal" fracture of the pubic ramus (B) is characteristic of lateral compression injuries. (Reprinted with permission from Young and Burgess.[11])

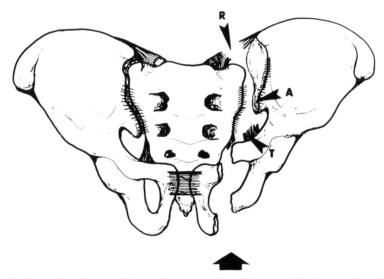

Figure 13–8. Vertical shear fracture. The injury force vector (arrow) is in a vertical plane, causing a shear injury to the hemipelvis. The pubic rami usually fractures anteriorly, and posterior instability is through either the sacrum, the joint, or the posterior iliac wing. The fracture lines are vertical and displacement is cephalad. The posterior (R) and anterior (A) ligaments can be disrupted, as well as the sacrospinous— sacrotuberous ligaments (T). (Reprinted with permission from Young and Burgess.[11])

vertical shear injuries, and 14% had complex patterns. The importance of the ability of the trauma team to identify quickly and classify the pelvic fracture is emphasized by the relationship between severe hemorrhage and visceral injury, and the degree and mechanism of pelvic disruption (Table 13–2). Dalal et al[9] found that type III AP compression patients had a significantly higher total fluid requirement than type III lateral compression injury patients. Type III AP compression patients were predisposed to a high incidence of circulatory shock (67%), adult respiratory distress syndrome (ARDS) (18.5%), sepsis (59%), and death (37%). A difference in the cause of mortality was also noted between the two injury pattern groups. Whereas the lateral compression deaths had a highly significant increase in the incidence of associated brain injury, AP compression deaths tended to have combined visceral injuries with high volume requirements. Although the lateral compression injury was more common in their series, the AP compression patients had a higher mortality because of the increased incidence of severe organ injury.

PELVIC FRACTURES

Acute Management

The morbidity and mortality of multiple trauma patients have been significantly lessened over the past decade, in part, because of the combined realization of both the trauma surgeon and the orthopedic surgeon that early, aggressive stabilization of major fractures positively affects pulmonary function, blood product requirements, and incidence of late sepsis.[15–18] The trend to eliminate requirements for skeletal traction, early mobilization of patients, and emphasis on the importance of the "upright chest" attitude of the post-trauma patient are the current expectations of the trauma surgeon and the goals of the orthopedic fracture surgeon.

Bone[16] reported a statistically significant higher incidence of pulmonary insufficiency, intensive care unit (ICU) days required, and hospitalization costs in trauma patients with injury severity scores greater than 18 who had stabilization of their femoral shaft fractures

Table 13–2   Classification and Complications of Pelvic Fractures*

	OCCURRENCE (%)		
	SEVERE HEMORRHAGE	BLADDER RUPTURE	URETHRA LESION
Lateral compression fractures			
Type I	0.5	4.0	2.0
Type II	36.0	7.0	0.0
Type III	60.0	20.0	20.0
AP compression fractures			
Type I	1.0	8.0	12.0
Type II	28.0	11.0	23.0
Type III	53.0	14.0	36.0
Vertical shear fractures	75.0	15.0	25.0
Mixed patterns	58.0	16.0	21.0

*Reprinted with permission from Young and Burgess.[11]

delayed beyond 48 hours. Johnson et al,[18] likewise, found a fivefold increase in the incidence of ARDS in patients treated with delayed fixation of their femoral fractures. Although major studies on the effects of aggressive stabilization of fractures are based on long bone injury, transference of the general principle to patients with unstable pelvic fractures should be allowed. Recent data from Latenser et al[31] indicate that this extrapolation is indeed valid.

Conservative management of a patient with an unstable pelvic fracture, and associated head and/or abdominal/thoracic injuries using traction and/or pelvic sling, is difficult. Ipsilateral traction to the hemipelvis, with or without a pelvic sling, restricts the patient to a recumbent position. Elevation of the head of the bed to relieve increased intracranial pressure or for increased pulmonary function is often required. Elimination of motion at the fracture site cannot be obtained. Positioning in the bed, transfer to gurneys for CT, angiography, or operating room visits will cause shifts in the unstable pelvic fracture, initiating additional bleeding and pain, thus increasing the requirements for blood products and analgesic support. Analgesia further depresses the pulmonary efforts.

The benefits of immediate reduction and stabilization of unstable pelvic fractures are:

1. Limits blood loss by stabilizing the fracture and the organizing retro-peritoneal hematoma, and by decreasing the potential volume of the retroperitoneal space[14]
2. Protects the adjacent neurovascular structure and soft tissues from additional injury
3. Decreases the patient's pain and, therefore, the analgesic requirements
4. Potentiates the efforts of the ICU team by creating a mobile patient capable of an "upright chest" position.

Our algorithm for the treatment of pelvic fractures is presented in Table 13–3.

Hemorrhage

Hemorrhage is the leading cause of death in patients with pelvic fractures, accounting for 60% of the mortality. Only 20% of the hemorrhagic deaths, however, are associated with major vessel injury.[2] Huittinen and Slatis[7] determined in postmortem studies that the source of bleeding in pelvic fractures was usually from small and medium caliber vessels and the cancellous bone. Most of the blood loss, however, probably originates from injury to the pelvic venous plexus. These factors, and the rich collateral circulation of the pelvic region, make standard operative approaches to control hemorrhage futile in most cases.[3] An accepted protocol for the evaluation and treatment of hemorrhage secondary to pelvic fractures has evolved, based on the merits of retroperitoneal tamponade, fracture stabilization, and selective arteriography and embolization.[3,5,6,20]

Trunkey et al[10] first attempted to identify the subset of patients prone to hemorrhage based on the fracture pattern. These efforts continue,[3,9,12] and have been successful in identifying that subset of patients that should undergo rapid diagnostic and therapeutic intervention prior to the onset of massive transfusion-associated coagulopathy. The subset includes type III AP and lateral compression and the vertical shear injuries. Cryer et al[12] showed, with a 90% confidence level, that 50 to 69% of these unstable pelvic fractures will require 4 U or more of blood and that 30 to 40% will require 10 U or more.

Table 13–3   Pelvic Fracture: Treatment Algorithm*

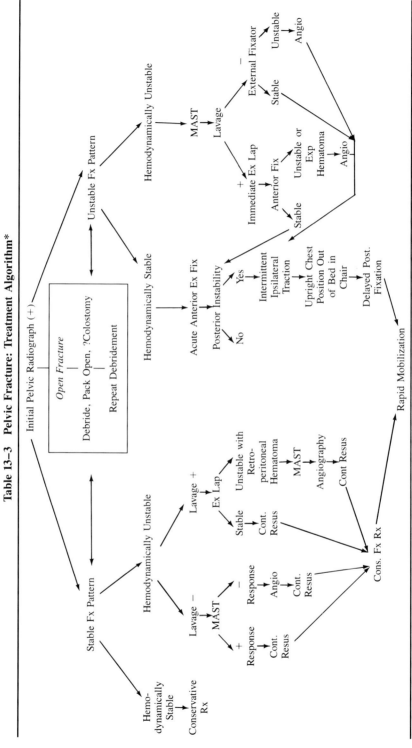

*Fx: fixation; Rx: treatment; MAST: Military Antishock Trousers; Ex: exterior; Lap: laparotomy; Cont: continuous; Resus: resuscitation; Exp: expanding; Angio: angiography; Post: posterior.

Initial review of the admission AP pelvic radiograph provides the diagnosis of the unstable pelvic fracture patient, that is, the patient at risk (Table 13–2). The patient's admission vital signs validate the extent of the hemorrhagic state. Naam et al[8] reported a 3% mortality in pelvic fracture patients who were normotensive on admission compared with a 38% mortality for patients with hypotension. The application of Military Antishock Trousers (MAST) is defined by most authors[3,6,8] as the first line of therapy in hypotensive pelvic fracture patients. MAST serve to stabilize the fracture and to increase the intra-abdominal and retroperitoneal pressure, assisting the tamponade of bleeding veins and small caliber arteries. Extended use of MAST, however, in the hypotensive patient can result in the development of compartment syndromes in the lower extremities,[32] and fasciotomies or the treatment of myoglobinuria may be required. Other sites of bleeding must be excluded. Most authors agree that a grossly positive peritoneal lavage requires immediate exploration. An external fixator should be applied to the pelvis at the same surgical procedure. Continual blood loss or visualization of an expanding retroperitoneal hematoma at celiotomy requires an angiographic examination.

A patient with an equivocal or a negative lavage who requires replacement of 6 U of blood requires an angiographic evaluation.[33] Some surgeons support application of external fixation prior to angiography to stabilize the pelvis, the hematoma, and the therapeutic arterial embolus, if required.[6,8,14,20]

External fixation of the pelvis and limitation of the potential hematoma volume by reduction of the pelvis has been successful in reducing blood requirements in most large centers. Reduction of the fracture decreases the osseous bleeding by immobilizing and approximating the cancellous surfaces and provides a tamponade effect to the retro-peritoneal hemorrhage by increasing the interstitial tissue pressure. Rubash and Mears[34] reported a 1.5 liter intrapelvic volume in a normal pelvis. The volume increased to 3 and 6 liters with diastasis of the pubic symphysis of 3 and 6 cm respectively. Reimer reduced the mortality rate from 22 to 8% with the use of an external fixator.[14] Edwards et al[13] reported that an 8 U blood requirement during 8 hours prior to the use of external fixation in his series was reduced to 2 U in the 20 hours following the application of external fixation. Moreno et al[6] found that the MAST were successful in controlling hemorrhage in 71% of their patients and that the external fixator was successful in 95% of the cases. A reduction in blood loss from 7.4 to 3.7 U was recognized with use of the external fixator.

Continued, unexplained blood loss, despite fracture stabilization, mandates emergency selective angiography. In 63 patients referred for angiographic studies, Kam et al[4] found 123 arterial injuries in 49 patients. The superior gluteal artery was the most frequently injured, followed by the internal pudendal, the obturator, and the lateral sacral arteries. Bleeding was most common from the internal pudendal. Mucha and Farnell[33] reported that angiography with embolization was successful in 86% of their patients.

Early recognition of the patient at risk, maximization of physiologic tamponade efforts by MAST application and external fixator, and early use of selective angiography are key elements in managing hemodynamically unstable pelvic fracture patients (Table 13–3).

OPEN PELVIC FRACTURES

Four percent of pelvic fractures are open. Uncontrolled hemorrhage and infection contribute to the significant mortality associated with this injury. Blood loss in open fracture patients is significantly higher than in closed fracture patients because of decompression and loss of the tamponade effect on the retroperitoneal hematoma. Most series report a high energy mechanism of injury, skewed to motorcycle and pedestrian accidents. Rothenberger et al[35] reported a 50% mortality rate in their open pelvic fracture patients, compared with 10% for closed fracture patients. Of the patients in their series, 57% were pedestrians; 27% had associated major vessel injury, contrasted to 0.3% of the closed fracture patients. This series predated the general use of MAST and selective angiography. Perry[36] reported a 42% mortality rate in his open fractures, in contrast to a 10.3% rate in the closed fractures. Recent mortality rates remain high with Govender et al[37] and Hanson et al[38] reporting mortality rates of 25% and 30%, respectively.

Utilizing a systematic approach to care of the open pelvic fracture patient, the following major facets are important:

1.   Control of hemorrhage
2.   Treatment of soft tissue wounds
3.   Recognition and treatment of associated injuries
4.   Treatment of the pelvic fracture

Richardson et al[39] reported a survival rate of 94.5% in 37 patients. The series emphasized angiography and embolization for uncontrolled hemorrhage. Wounds were aggressively explored and debrided, packed open, and serially reexplored and debrided of necrotic tissue at follow-up surgeries. As recommended by Maull et al[40] and Rothenberger et al,[35,41] a diverting colostomy was performed on all patients with bowel injury, buttock or perineal wounds. In contrast to current practice, however, these series treated the pelvic fractures conservatively, using bed rest and pelvic straps.

Early Fracture Stabilization

Fixation of the pelvic fracture is divided into two phases: acute emergent stabilization and delayed elective internal fixation. The immediate goals of the orthopedic trauma surgeon in a patient with an unstable pelvic fracture are to assist in the control of the hemorrhage by rapidly stabilizing the pelvis and limiting the volume of the retroperitoneal hematoma. Acute stabilization of the pelvis in a patient with multiple injuries also positively contributes to the ICU efforts to provide postresuscitation care by allowing safe mobilization of the patient and an "upright chest" patient attitude. These goals must be achieved within the constraints of the acute trauma setting. The fixation procedure should be a rapid, simple surgical procedure that avoids decompression or potential contamination of the retroperitoneal hematoma. External fixation is the procedure of choice for the acute stabilization of the unstable pelvic fracture.

External Fixation

Unstable pelvic disruptions without a significant vertical shear component or disruption of the posterior SI ligaments can usually be managed with an anterior external fixation frame. AP compression or lateral compression injuries without complete disruption of the SI joint require simple frames consisting of groups of two to three 5 mm pins placed in the anterior iliac wings and connected by means of articulating couplings and bars, following closed fracture reduction.[42] Fracture reduction maneuvers are opposite the injury vector.

More rigid frames have been devised in order to attempt to control injuries with complete disruption of the SI joint or vertical shear fractures.[43] However, no anterior frame can stabilize these severe pelvic disruptions completely.[23] They do provide sufficient stability to allow the patient to be mobilized to a chair, especially when combined with ipsilateral traction in patients with posterior pelvic instability.

External Fixation with Traction

In addition to the anterior external fixation frame, skeletal traction should be applied to the ipsilateral lower extremity to control proximal migration of the hemipelvis in patients with posterior pelvic instability. This should be maintained until the fracture has healed or until definitive internal fixation can be carried out. The traction, however, should not be allowed to interfere with patient care. It can be intermittent and maintained with the patient in a sitting position, either in bed or in a chair.

External Fixation Combined with Internal Fixation

In limited situations, internal and external fixation of the pelvis are combined in the acute trauma patient. The external fixator provides anterior stability, but does little to control either posterior or cephalad migration of the hemipelvis, with gross posterior instability.[23,43] Posterior iliac wing fractures, sacral fractures, and SI joint dislocations can be addressed acutely in selected patients,[23] with the anterior pelvic instability managed by external fixation (Fig. 13–9). Internal fixation should be avoided in patients who are hemodynamically unstable for fear of decompressing the tamponade effect of the retroperitoneal hematoma. Immediate internal fixation should also be avoided in patients with bladder injury or who require a diverting colostomy because of the significant risk of infection.

Acute plating of the pubic symphysis should be considered in patients with an anterior compression injury with disruption of the pubis who are undergoing an uncontaminated exploration, and the pubis could be easily approached without excessive extension of the celiotomy incision.[44,45] In patients with associated posterior instability, an external fixator is also applied, until the posterior pelvis can undergo reconstruction.[43,45]

IMMEDIATE INTERNAL FIXATION

Immediate, definitive internal fixation of the unstable pelvic fracture is avoided by most authors because of anticipated hemorrhagic or infectious complications. Recently, however, Goldstein et al[46] reported on a series of patients who underwent immediate open reduction and internal fixation for unstable pelvic fractures. In this series of 15 patients, seven underwent this surgery within 24 hours of injury. In most of the cases, anterior and posterior internal fixation was carried out simultaneously. Preoperative angiography and embolization were used to help control hemorrhage in five of the patients. In this small uncontrolled series, early surgery appeared to be beneficial, or, at least, not detrimental to the patient. A controlled, prospective series evaluating immediate versus delayed open reduction of acute unstable pelvic fractures will be necessary to validate the advantages of this approach.

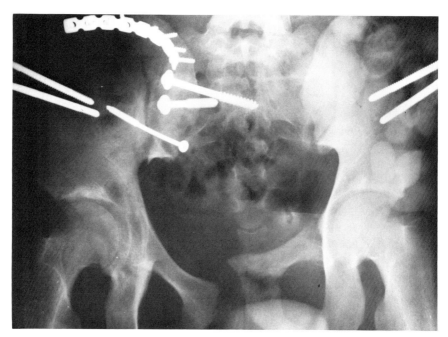

Figure 13–9.   A hemodynamically stable patient with anterior and complex posterior pelvic fractures was treated immediately with open reduction and fixation of the posterior iliac wing and SI joint injury. An anterior external fixation frame was added to neutralize the anterior instability.

Spica Cast Application

Cotler et al[47] reported on the immediate application of a bilateral hip spica cast incorporating femoral or tibial skeletal traction pins as a means of reducing and stabilizing pelvic ring disruptions. This method seemed to assist in the control of hemorrhage from the fracture but recumbency was required. Increased pulmonary complications were noted in the patients.

DELAYED DEFINITIVE INTERNAL FIXATION

The goals of delayed open reduction and internal fixation of unstable pelvic fractures are to prevent late morbidity related to malreduction of the pelvis and to prevent prolonged recumbency. In a postmortem study, Bucholz[27] found that anatomic reduction of the SI joint was difficult to obtain because of soft tissue interposition in the joint space. Most authors have found that even if an anatomic reduction can be obtained initially, unstable injuries undergo migration of either the SI joint or the fracture.[23,48] Tile[23] found that the most common unsatisfactory results were in patients with sacroiliac joint dislocations. Chronic pain was present in 60% of the patients. Edwards et al[13] reported suboptimal late results using external fixation alone for unstable pelvic fractures. Although 60% of posterosuperior displacements were reduced, only 20% were maintained. Prolonged supplemental traction improved ultimate displacement by only 10%. Edwards et al concluded that although the external fixation did assist in obtaining hemodynamic stability, significantly decrease patient pain, and provide a means for rapid mobilization, the late orthopedic clinical results were no better than those reported for series predating the use of external fixation. In their series, 48% of patients had late SI joint pain, 45% had sitting discomfort, and 52% had leg length discrepancy of 1 cm or greater. Fifty-two percent of patients were unable to run, and 36% of patients restricted their former daily activities.

Open anatomic reduction with stable internal fixation, supplemented with fusion of the SI joint should provide the best orthopedic clinical result. In most centers, definite open reduction and fixation of the unstable pelvic fracture is delayed until the patient and the retroperitoneal hematoma are stable, usually at 7 to 10 days.[44,49] Major complications associated with delayed pelvic fixation are infection of the operative site and retroperitoneal hematoma. Optimization of all patient parameters should be emphasized prior to the planned surgery. The patient's nutritional profile requires specific attention.[50] Surgical procedures should be planned to avoid incorporation of the external fixation pins in the operative field because of the risk of bacterial contamination.

Fixation for Disrupted Sacroiliac Joint

Sacroiliac joint disruptions can be repaired through either an anterior ilioinguinal approach or by means of a posterior approach. The posterior surgical approach is simple and direct; obtaining a reduction is perhaps easier, but fixation is technically more demanding. Good stable fixation can be obtained by passing 6.5 mm cancellous screws from the posterior iliac wing through the SI joint into the ala of the sacrum and first sacral vertebral body.[14,23] C-arm image intensification control is recommended to prevent malplacement of the screws into the neural canal, neural foramina, or from protruding out anteriorly. Posterior plates and screws, as well as transsacral bars, have been used successfully to stabilize SI joint disruptions, particularly in patients with bilateral SI joint disruptions. The posterior approach to the SI joint is performed with the anterior external fixator in place. The fixator is maintained for 8 to 12 weeks postoperatively.

The anterior surgical approach to the SI joint is slightly more demanding. While obtaining a reduction may be somewhat more difficult, internal fixation using reconstruction plates and screws is relatively straightforward. Compression plates are used to obtain fixation. If an external fixator is in place, it should be removed and the pin tracts allowed to heal prior to the use of the anterior approach.

Because of the likelihood of eventual failure of fixation, as well as the probability of arthritis developing as a late sequelae to SI joint disruption, many authors recommend debridement of the articular cartilage from the SI joint. This is performed with or without cancellous bone grafting to attempt arthrodesis of the joint at the time of internal fixation.[44,51,52]

Fixation for Sacral Fractures

Most sacral fractures requiring open reduction and internal fixation are adequately stabilized by either transsacral compression rods, bolts, or contoured reconstruction plates and screws.[14,23,44]

Fixation for Disruptions of the Symphysis Pubis

Disruption of the symphysis pubis with spread of less than 3 cm, not accompanied by significant posterior disruption, usually improves with ambulation and does not require fixation. Disruptions of the symphysis pubis requiring repair can be accomplished either through a low Pfannenstiel transverse incision or a short midline vertical incision. Single or double plates and screws placed over the superior or anterior aspect of the symphysis are utilized.[14,23,44,45] The symphysis pubis often needs to be repaired in conjunction with repair of a disrupted sacroiliac joint or with the reconstruction of a complex acetabular fracture. If amenable, an ilioinguinal approach can be used to repair both the symphysis and acetabulum, symphysis and SI joint, or all three. Associated complex acetabular fractures often require an extensive surgical approach that can address the reconstruction of the SI joint, the pubis, and the acetabulum.[14,23,53]

Fixation for Iliac Wing Fractures

Fractures of the iliac wing that are components of unstable pelvic ring injuries can be approached either internally, by means of an ilioinguinal incision, or externally by an incision along the iliac crest. These fractures are easily fixed using plates and lag screws.

Fixation for Pubic Rami Fractures

Fractures of the pubic rami, which occur as components of pelvic ring disruptions, ordinarily heal rapidly and do not require surgical repair. However, in cases that require stabilization in conjunction with repair of posterior disruption, or reconstruction of acetabular fractures, or in cases of pelvic ring malunion, all or part of an ilioinguinal approach is required. Screws or plates and screws provide fixation.

LONG-TERM RESULTS

Unstable pelvic fractures are the result of high-energy trauma. Patients sustaining these injuries must be advised early in their clinical course that a mild to moderate degree of permanent to partial disability will result despite all efforts. Neurologic lesions are defined at the time of the accident. Late pelvic pain and leg length discrepancy are directly related to the quality of fracture reduction and later to the stability of the symphysis and the SI joint. Internal fixation of unstable pelvic fractures yielded significantly better results in patients reported by Mears and Rubash.[14] Kellam et al[44] reported a similar experience, but recognized a 25% wound infection rate. Often, the patient's clinical status prevents early reconstruction surgery. After the patient recovers, disabilities can be addressed.

Pelvic nonunions or delayed unions can be successfully treated with fixation and bone grafting.[54] SI joint pain can be relieved with a fusion.

SUMMARY

Early recognition of the patient at risk for hemorrhage and associated visceral injury, prompt resuscitation with aggressive use of external fixation and selective angiography, treatment of associated injuries, and rapid mobilization of the patient to prevent pulmonary complications will continue to provide excellent clinical results and lower mortality rates for patients with unstable pelvic fractures. Carefully planned delayed reconstruction surgery will minimize the orthopedic morbidity associated with the injury.

REFERENCES

1. McMurtry R, Walton D, Dickinson D, Kellam J, Tile M: Pelvic disruption in the polytraumatized patient: A management protocol. *Clin Orthop* 1980;151:22–29.
2. Brown JJ, Green FL, McMillin RD: Vascular injuries associated with pelvic fractures. *Am Surg* 1984;50:150–154.
3. Flint LM, Brown A, Richardson JD, Polk HC: Definitive control of bleeding from severe pelvic fractures. *Ann Surg* 1979;189:709–716.
4. Kam J, Jackson H, Ben-Menachem Y: Vascular injuries in blunt pelvic trauma. *Radiol Clin North Am* 1981;19:171–186.
5. Maull KI, Sachatello CR: Current management of pelvic fractures: A combined surgical-angiographic approach to hemorrhage. *South Med J* 1976;69:1285–1289.
6. Moreno C, Moore EE, Rosenberger A, Cleveland HC: Hemorrhage associated with major pelvic fracture: A multispecialty challenge. *J Trauma* 1986;26:987–993.
7. Huittinen, V, Slatis, P: Postmortem angiography and dissection of the hypogastric artery in pelvic fractures. *Surgery* 1973;73:454–462.
8. Naam NJ, Brown WH, Hurd R, Burdge RE, Kaminski DL: Major pelvic fractures. *Arch Surg* 1983;118:610–615.
9. Dalal SA, Burgess AR, Siegal JH, Young JW, Brumback RJ, Poka A, Dunham CM, Gens D, Bathon H: Pelvic fracture in multiple trauma: Classification by mechanism is key to pattern of organ injury, resuscitative requirements and outcome. *J Trauma* 1989;29:981–1002.
10. Trunkey DD, Chapman MW, Lim RC, Dunphy JE: Management of pelvic fractures in blunt trauma injury. *J Trauma* 1974;11:912–923.
11. Young JW, Burgess AR: Radiologic Management of Pelvic Ring Fractures: Systematic Radiographic Diagnosis. Baltimore: Urban and Schwarzenberg, 1987.
12. Cryer HM, Miller FB, Evers BM, Rouben LB, Seligson, DL: Pelvic fracture classification: Correlation with hemorrhage. *J Trauma* 1988;28:973–980.
13. Edwards CC, Meier PJ, Browner BD, Freedman MA, Ackley SM: Results treating 50 unstable pelvic injuries using primary external fixation. *Orthop Trans* 1985;9:434.
14. Mears DC, Rubash HE: Pelvic and Acetabular Fractures. Thorofare, NJ: Slack, 1986.
15. Gylling SF, Ward RE, Holcroft JW, Chapman MW: Immediate external fixation of unstable pelvic fractures. *Am J Surg* 1985;150:721–724.
16. Bone LB: Prospective randomized study of femoral fracture: Early versus delayed stabilization and pulmonary insufficiency. *Orthop Trans* 1987;11:490.
17. Bone LB, Bucholz R: The management of fractures in the patient with multiple trauma. *J Bone Joint Surg* 1986;68:945–949.
18. Johnson KD, Cadambi A, Seibert GB: Incidence of adult respiratory distress syndrome in patients with multiple musculoskeletal injuries: Effect of early operative stabilization of fractures. *J Trauma* 1985;25:375–377.
19. Colapinto V: Trauma to the pelvis: Urethral injury. *Clin Orthop* 1980;151:46–55.
20. Cowley RA, Dunham CM (ed): *Shock Trauma/Critical Care Manual: Initial Assessment and Management.* Baltimore: University Park Press, 1982.
21. Winquist R, Mayo K: ORIF of unstable ring fractures. Presented at the Orthopedic Trauma Association Meeting, Dallas, October 1988.
22. Gilloti A, Rhodes M, Luckie J: Utility of routine pelvic x-ray during blunt trauma resuscitation. *J Trauma* 1988;28:1570–1573.
23. Tile M: *Fractures of the Pelvis and Acetabulum.* Baltimore: Williams & Wilkins, 1984.

24. Gill K, Bucholz RW: The role of computerized tomographic scanning in the evaluation of major pelvic fractures. *J Bone Joint Surg* 1984;66:34–39.

25. Peters P, Bucholz R: Stress testing of pelvic ring fractures. Presented at the Orthopedic Trauma Association Meeting, Dallas, October 1988.

26. Pennal GF, Tile M, Waddel JP, Garside H: Pelvic disruption: Assessment and classification. *Clin Orthop* 1980;151:12–21.

27. Bucholz RW: The pathological anatomy of Malgaigne fracture—dislocations of the pelvis. *J Bone Joint Surg* 1981;63:400–404.

28. Young JW, Burgess AR, Brumback RJ, Poka A: Lateral compression fractures of the pelvis: The importance of plain radiographs in the diagnosis and surgical management. *Skel Radiol* 1986;15:103–109.

29. Bosse MJ, Poka A, Reinert CM, Brumback RJ, Bathon H, Burgess AR: Preoperative angiographic assessment of the superior gluteal artery in acetabular fractures requiring extensile surgical exposures. *J Orthop Trauma* 1989;2:303–307.

30. Smith K, Ben-Menachem Y, Duke JH, Hill GL: The superior gluteal: An artery at risk in blunt pelvic trauma. *J Trauma* 1976;16:273–279.

31. Latenser BA, Gentilello LM, Tarver AA, et al: Improved outcome with early fixation of skeletally unstable pelvic fractures. *J Trauma* 1991;31:28–31.

32. Williams TM, Knopp R, Ellyson JH: Compartment syndrome after anti-shock trouser use without lower extremity trauma. *J Trauma* 1982;22:595–597.

33. Mucha P, Farnell MB: Analysis of pelvic fracture management. *J Trauma* 1984;24:379–386.

34. Rubash HE, Mears DC: External and internal fixation of the pelvis. In AAOS Instructional Course Lecture. St. Louis: CV Mosby, 1983;32:329.

35. Rothenberger D, Velasco R, Strate R, Fischer RP, Perry, JF: Open pelvic fractures: A lethal injury. *J Trauma*, 1978;18:184–187.

36. Perry JF: Pelvic open fractures. *Clin Orthop* 1980;151:41–45.

37. Govender S, Sham A, Single B: Open pelvic fractures. *Injury* 1990;21:373–376.

38. Hanson PB, Milne JC, Chapman MW: Open fractures of the pelvis: Review of 43 cases. *J Bone Joint Surg* 1991;73-B:325–329.

39. Richardson JD, Harty J, Amin M, Flint LM: Open pelvic fractures. *J Trauma* 1982;22:533–538.

40. Maull KI, Sachatello CR, Ernst CB: The deep perineal laceration—an injury frequently associated with open pelvic fractures: A need for aggressive surgical management. *J Trauma* 1977;17:685–696.

41. Rothenberger DA, Fischer RP, Strate RG, Velasco R, Perry JF: The mortality associated with pelvic fractures. *Surgery* 1978;84:356–359.

42. Slatis P, Karaharju EO: External fixation of unstable pelvic fractures: Experience in 22 patients treated with a trapezoid compression frame. *Clin Orthop* 1980;151:73–79.

43. Mears DC, Fu FH: Modern concepts of external skeletal fixation of the pelvis. *Clin Orthop* 1980;151:65–72.

44. Kellam JF, McMurtry RY, Paley F, Tile M: The unstable pelvic fracture: Operative treatment. *Orthop Clin North Am* 1987;18:25–41.

45. Lange RH, Hansen ST: Pelvic ring disruptions with symphysis pubis diastasis: Indications, techniques and limitations of anterior internal fixation. *Clin Orthop* 1985;201:130–137.

46. Goldstein A, Phillips R, Salafani SJ, Scalea T, Duncan A, Goldstein J, Panetta, Shaftan G: Early open reduction and internal fixation of the disrupted pelvic ring. *J Trauma* 1986;26:325–333.

47. Cotler HB, Lamont JG, Hansen ST: Immediate spica casting for pelvic fractures. *J Orthop Trauma* 1988;2:222–228.

48. Wild JJ, Hanson GW, Tullos HS: Unstable fractures of the pelvis treated by external fixation. *J Bone Joint Surg* 1982;64:1010–1019.

49. Browner BD, Cole JD, Graham JM, Bondurant FJ, Nunchuck-Burns SK, Cotler HB: Delayed posterior internal fixation of unstable pelvic fractures. *J Trauma* 1987;27:998–1005.

50. Jensen JE, Jensen TG, Smith TK, Johnson DA, Duduck SJ: Nutrition in orthopedic surgery. *J Bone Joint Surg* 1982;64:1263–1271.

51. Simpson LA, Waddell JP, Leighton RK, Kellam JF, Tile M: Anterior approach and stabilization of the disrupted sacroiliac joint. *J Trauma* 1987;27:1332–1338.

52. Gershuni D, O'Hara R: Primary fusion in the treatment of sacroiliac disruption. Presented at the Orthopedic Trauma Association Meeting, Baltimore, November 1987.

53. Reinert CM, Bosse JJ, Poka A, Schacherer TG, Brumback RJ, Burgess AR: A modified extensile exposure for the treatment of complex or malunited acetabular fractures. *J Bone Joint Surg* 1988;70:329–337.

54. Pennal GF, Massiah KA: Nonunion and delayed union of fractures of the pelvis. *Clin Orthop* 1980;151:124–129.

14

Diaphragmatic Trauma

SCOTT B. FRAME, M.D., F.A.C.S.

The history of diaphragmatic injuries in the medical literature dates back to the original description by Sennertus in 1541.[1] He described the autopsy findings in a man who had sustained a penetrating chest wound 7 months prior to his death. The patient succumbed to a herniation of the stomach through a diaphragmatic defect secondary to the earlier trauma.

Ambrose Paré[2] receives credit for the next reports in the literature with descriptions of two patients. The first was an autopsy report in 1579 in which the cause of death was colonic strangulation in a diaphragmatic defect "no bigger than the tip of the little finger." This defect was the result of a bullet wound incurred 8 months earlier. Later Paré described the postmortem findings in a stonemason who died several months after blunt abdominal trauma. The cause of death in this patient was also gastric herniation.

The first report of antemortem diagnosis of traumatic diaphragmatic hernia is attributed to Bowditch in 1853.[3] He also included in this report a review of 83 autopsies from the literature. With these data he recommended specific criteria for the physical diagnosis of post-traumatic diaphragmatic hernia. His five criteria included: (1) immobility of the left thorax; (2) displacement of the area of cardiac dullness to the right; (3) absent breath sounds in the left hemithorax; (4) bowel sounds audible in the chest; and (5) tympany to percussion over the left thorax.

The first reported case of successful repair of a diaphragmatic injury dates to 1886.[4,5] Riolfi described the repair of a stab wound through the diaphragm, which contained herniated omentum.

These early reports highlight the natural history of undiagnosed and untreated diaphragmatic injuries. The rule is that a hollow viscus will eventually herniate through even very small defects, as dramatically pointed out by the findings in Paré's first patient. Therefore even the smallest injury cannot be taken for granted, and must be carefully sought for in the trauma patient. The diagnosis of these injuries is often difficult, and they may be overlooked during the trauma celiotomy unless the surgeon carries out a diligent inspection of the entire diaphragm.

The incidence of injuries to the diaphragm in penetrating trauma to the chest has been reported to be 10 to 15% in a series from San Antonio.[6,7] In the same series, when the

193

wound was anterior and below the nipple line, the incidence of diaphragmatic injury was 30%. Moore et al[8] observed in the Denver General Hospital population that 15% of patients with stab wounds and 46% of patients with gunshot wounds to the lower chest had associated intra-abdominal injuries with violation of the diaphragm. It has been estimated that 4.5% of patients requiring hospitalization for blunt multitrauma have a diaphragmatic tear.[9] In patients requiring celiotomy or thoracotomy for trauma, the incidence of injury to the diaphragm has been reported to be 5.8 to 8.0%.[10,11]

The signs and symptoms of diaphragmatic injury are subtle and nonspecific. They are often overshadowed by other injuries in the multitrauma patient.[12] For this reason, it is mandatory that the surgeon caring for the trauma patient maintain a high degree of suspicion for the possibility of the presence of diaphragmatic trauma.

ANATOMY

The diaphragm is a large dome-shaped sheet of skeletal muscle separating the thorax from the abdomen. The undersurface of the diaphragm is invested with parietal peritoneum, the posterior attachments are along the lumbar vertebra, and therefore it is included in the structures comprising the retroperitoneum. It primarily functions as a muscle of respiration and is noteworthy for its resistance to fatigue. Diaphragmatic action accounts for two thirds of the tidal volume in the erect adult.[13] Loss of function of one leaf of the diaphragm results in a reduction in pulmonary function of 25 to 50%.[14]

Embryologically, the diaphragm is formed from the fusion of the septum transversum, the pleuroperitoneal and pleurocardial folds, the dorsal mesentery, and a mesodermal rim from the lateral body wall.[15]

The architecture of the diaphragm consists of a central tendon surrounded by radially arranged muscle bundles attached to the lateral chest wall. The posterior attachments of the diaphragm are on the periosteal surfaces of the first, second, and third lumbar vertebrae. The anterior attachments are to the lowermost sternum at the junction with the xiphoid. From this central attachment, the muscle fans out laterally, attaching to the internal surfaces of the lower ribs. The lateral attachments extend from the 12th rib posteriorly to the sixth rib anteriorly. The dome of the right diaphragm may extend up to the fourth intercostal space and the left dome to the fifth intercostal space at full expiration (Fig. 14–1).

The two halves of the diaphragm are enervated separately by the phrenic nerve on each side. The phrenic nerve arises from the third, fourth, and fifth cervical nerve roots and runs through the posterolateral mediastinum on the surface of the pericardium. The phrenic nerves insert into the diaphragm at the junction of the pericardium and the central tendon, and fan out radially over the superior surface in a "crow's foot" pattern. Blood supply to the diaphragm consists of central vessels that run with the phrenic nerves, inferiorly by direct branches from the aorta, and peripherally by branches from the intercostal arteries.

The diaphragm is able to move through a 10 cm vertical arc during labored breathing and 3 to 5 cm during normal respiration. It is therefore difficult to determine the exact position of the diaphragm at any given point in time. Penetrating injuries of the lower chest below the level of the fourth intercostal space must be suspected of having caused trauma to the diaphragm. Blunt trauma to the abdomen may also increase intra-abdominal pressure to the point where a blowout injury of the diaphragm may occur.

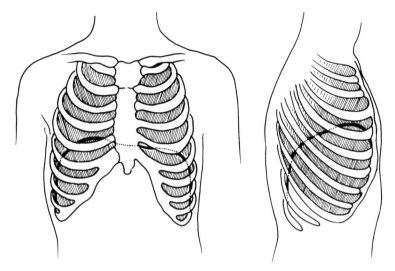

Figure 14–1. Limits of diaphragmatic excursion at full expiration.

PATHOPHYSIOLOGY

Blunt Trauma

Blunt abdominal trauma that results in a rapid rise in intra-abdominal pressure may cause rupture of one or both of the diaphragmatic leaflets. When the pressure within the abdomen rises rapidly enough and high enough, a large pressure gradient results between the thorax and the abdomen. This instantaneous gradient results in a burst injury to the diaphragm. The tears may involve one or both leaflets and usually begin at the central tendon and radiate posteriorly and laterally. Tears secondary to blunt trauma have been described in all portions of the diaphragm. Most commonly, the left hemidiaphragm has been reportedly involved with the greatest frequency, with 79% to 20% left:right figures quoted in a review of several series from the 1980s.[16] This tenet has been questioned.[17] The routinely held theory has been that the liver "protects" the right side from damage. What possibly occurs is the liver hides the defect by, in essence, "plugging" the hole that is created. The possibility is great that both hemidiaphragms are involved with similar frequency, but that the right-sided injuries are less commonly diagnosed and, due to the protective influence of the liver, cause fewer late complications. Tears have been reported in every portion of the diaphragm,[18] even injuries confined to the central portion with isolated herniation into the pericardium.[19,20] Bilateral tears and complex unilateral tears with extension into the pericardial surface have also been reported.[21]

The most common scenario for mechanism of injury is a high-speed deceleration accident with a restrained passenger. The victim is thrown forward against the lap belt. When the lap belt is improperly applied, riding high over the abdomen, the forces from the impact are transferred directly to the abdominal cavity. A properly applied lap belt should ride over the iliac crests where forces are dissipated to the bony structures of the pelvis. Other mechanisms include falls, blows to the abdomen (i.e., assaults or horse kicks), and crush injuries resulting in compressive forces to the abdominal cavity.

Direct injury to the diaphragm from rib fractures may also occur in blunt trauma. These injuries may result in severe lacerations, which tend to bleed more profusely than the burst injuries. They are also usually associated with severe pulmonary contusion on the ipsilateral side. Hollow viscus perforation from the protruding rib fragments is rare, but lacerations of the underlying liver and spleen may occur with attendant profuse hemorrhage.

Penetrating Wounds

Obviously, the most common mechanisms of injury are gunshot and stab wounds. However, missile fragments, material thrown up by power equipment, and debris from explosions may also be the wounding agents resulting in injury to the diaphragm. The classic scenario in penetrating trauma is that of the downward directed stab wound to the lower anterior chest. As previously stated, the diaphragm may rise to the level of the fourth intercostal space, so any anterior chest wound below the nipple line must be suspected of having associated diaphragmatic injury.

Injuries secondary to penetrating trauma usually are smaller lacerations, 1 to 2 cm in length. The injuries are normally smaller than the large rents produced by the blunt burst injuries. A pressure gradient normally exists across the diaphragm. The thorax maintains a median negative pressure, whereas the abdominal cavity has a constant positive pressure. This positive pressure in the abdomen normally is 7 to 20 cm H_2O,[22] but may reach 150 to 200 mmHg during maximal muscle contraction.[23] The existence of this continual pressure gradient, which is exacerbated by exertion and coughing, leads to a situation in which intra-abdominal contents tend to be forced up into the defect. It is rare for even the smallest of injuries to seal due to the presence of this pressure gradient. Clearly, the natural history of any diaphragmatic perforation is as just described, and no injury, no matter how seemingly insignificant, should be considered safe from future complications.[24,25] All injuries must be carefully sought after and repaired when found.

General Considerations

The immediate complications of diaphragmatic disruption are derangements in cardiopulmonary function. The long-term sequelae are gastrointestinal. Hemodynamic instability may be initially present. Even though bleeding may be profuse from the torn edges of the defect in the diaphragm, it is rarely massive. Hypovolemic shock in these patients is usually secondary to blood loss from associated injuries, not from the diaphragmatic wound. The displacement of intra-abdominal organs into the thoracic cavity may interfere with respiratory function or cardiac ventricular filling, or both. Isolated rupture into the pericardial space may produce acute pericardial tamponade. As stated previously, the loss of one hemidiaphragm may result in a decrease in respiratory function of 25 to 50%. This decrease in the already stressed trauma patient may be sufficient to cause respiratory failure. Often, pulmonary contusions may be present due to the force of impact in blunt trauma, and both contusions and compression of lung parenchyma by displaced organs cause compromise in pulmonary function.

Gastrointestinal complications result from incarceration and strangulation of hollow viscus in the thoracic cavity. Rupture of the gastrointestinal (GI) tract into the chest leads to serious septic complications. Right hemidiaphragm injuries may lead to herniation of the liver and there are reports of hepatic coma secondary to herniation and torsion, with ischemia of the liver.[26]

DIAGNOSIS

Clinical Presentation

The signs and symptoms of acute diaphragmatic injury are nonspecific and usually are secondary to the associated injuries present. The history obtained from the prehospital personnel that significant forces were involved in the accident should also alert the clinician. The most common complaint has been said to be generalized abdominal pain,[27] a symptom that is not very helpful in the multitrauma patient.

The blunt trauma patient may have contusions over the chest and abdomen. Seat belt contusions over the abdomen, demonstrating that the lap belt had been improperly applied, should alert the examiner to the possibility of diaphragmatic disruption. Pelvic fractures, multiple extremity fractures, and multiple rib fractures are all indicative of trauma involving high-energy transfer to the patient and should raise the level of suspicion. As stated previously, hypovolemic shock is rarely a direct consequence of the diaphragmatic injury, but rather secondary to associated injuries. Exsanguinating hemorrhage into the thoracic cavity may occur from a severe hepatic or splenic injury that has herniated into the chest through a diaphragmatic tear. Occasionally, patients may present with tension hemithorax from herniated abdominal viscus, or pericardial tamponade from herniation into the pericardial sac or cardiac torsion through the diaphragmatic defect.

The location of penetrating wounds will give valuable indications as to whether or not the diaphragm may be involved. Entrance and exit wounds from gunshots give some information as to the possible missile tract and may indicate that the diaphragm has been traversed. As stated earlier, wounds over the lower anterior chest (below the nipple line) should be considered as potentially violating the diaphragm.

After the acute phase, if the patient has not had the injury diagnosed, he enters the interval or latent phase. This phase may last up to 2 or 3 years. This occurs if the patient does not have significant enough associated injuries to necessitate exploratory celiotomy, the diaphragmatic injury is missed at exploration, or the injury is not diagnosed by routine measures. The occult defect then runs its natural course, and the diagnosis is eventually made by serendipity or the patient develops obstruction in the herniated organs.

The patients in the latent phase are usually symptomatic.[21] They may present complaining of intermittent upper abdominal pain, a vague upper abdominal discomfort, nausea, or vomiting. Bernatz et al[21] reported frequent left shoulder pain, especially in the supine position. These authors cited an incidence in their patients of 50% GI complaints, 25% dyspnea or abnormal sensations in the chest, and 25% pain in the left upper abdomen or lower chest. These vague symptoms may lead the patient to seek medical aid and the diagnosis is commonly made on chest radiograph.

The patient may not seek medical attention for the minor symptoms, and, as we have seen, the natural course is for increasing amounts of intra-abdominal material to herniate into the chest. On the left side, this commonly consists of the stomach or colon, or both. The hollow viscus may become distended and then develop torsion and obstruction. When this occurs, the patient may experience severe, constant abdominal pain, nausea and vomiting, and dyspnea. When this stage is reached, a surgical emergency exists and immediate surgical intervention is mandatory to avoid strangulation, perforation, and death. When strangulation does occur, it will present within 3 years of the traumatic incident in 85% of cases.[28]

Diagnostic Techniques

Chest Radiography

The single most useful diagnostic maneuver in either the acute or latent phases is the chest radiograph (Figs. 14–2, 14–3, 14–4). The admitting film must be carefully examined for the subtle findings associated with diaphragmatic disruption. The findings that are considered highly suggestive or diagnostic of injury are unilateral elevation or an indistinct character to a hemidiaphragm; a mass, either solid or hollow, above the diaphragm; a hollow viscus present above the hepatic shadow on the right; free air beneath the diaphragm in a patient with a penetrating chest wound; mediastinal shift away from the affected side; or the nasogastric tube coiled above the diaphragm or present behind the cardiac silhouette. Other nonspecific abnormalities that should raise the level of suspicion are multiple rib fractures,

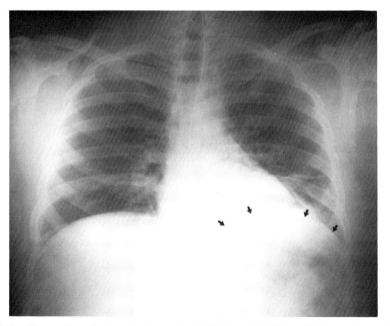

Figure 14–2.   Chest radiograph demonstrating gastric bubble above the left hemidiaphragm (arrows).

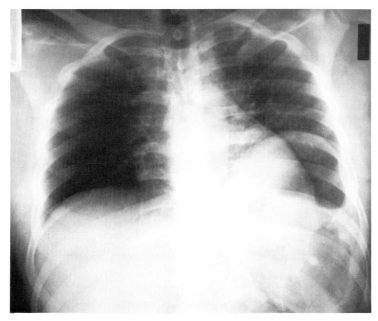

Figure 14–3. Chest radiograph of the same patient demonstrating progression of gastric herniation into the left chest.

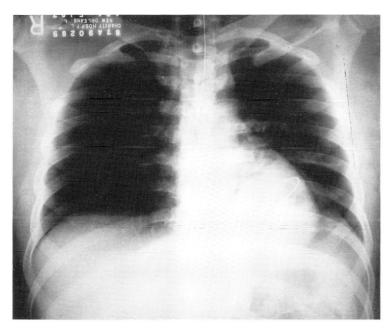

Figure 14–4. Chest radiograph after nasogastric tube insertion demonstrating tube coiled above the left hemidiaphragm.

especially of the lower ribs; hemothorax; pneumothorax; pulmonary contusion; or mediastinal widening.

Even though the chest radiograph is considered the best current diagnostic test, it is far from what we would consider an excellent study. Wise et al[29] reported a 36% incidence of normal chest films in patients with proven diaphragmatic injury from penetrating trauma. Waldschmidt and Laws[10] found in their series that 23% of films were read as normal, 60% were read as abnormal, and only 17% had findings interpreted as diagnostic of diaphragmatic disruption. Blunt trauma usually involves high-energy transfer to the patient and multisystem injury. The films were still only 50% suggestive or diagnostic of diaphragmatic injury. Twelve percent of the films were read as normal. In the acute setting the only view that is normally obtained is the anteroposterior film. This may account for the poor showing of the chest radiograph in the diagnostic arena. Subsequent erect posteroanterior and lateral views are usually more helpful in delineating diaphragmatic pathologic aspects.

Special Radiograph Studies

Special studies are rarely useful and may be dangerous to take the time to perform in the acute setting when the patient is critically ill. However, in the stable patient, contrast studies may provide valuable information in the patient with suspected diaphragmatic injury. Barium upper GI studies and barium enemas may demonstrate upward displacement of the stomach or herniated colon into the thoracic cavity. Since blunt diaphragmatic tears are often posterior in location, lateral views are essential in any contrast study to provide the maximum amount of anatomic information. Fluoroscopy with or without contrast medium can provide information on diaphragmatic motility. This test is especially useful during the latent phase. A paralyzed hemidiaphragm is strong evidence for diaphragmatic injury in the patient with a prior history of trauma.

Computed tomography (CT) of the abdomen and lower chest has been advocated by some as the diagnostic test of choice for diaphragmatic injury. Trunkey stated that CT was 100% accurate in diagnosing post-traumatic diaphragmatic hernia in a 1987 lecture in Britain.[30] However, others do not share his enthusiasm for the accuracy of this test. Small tears such as those produced by penetrating trauma may be easily missed and, if no organs are herniated through the defect, the lesion may also be overlooked. Recently, magnetic resonance imaging has been reported as another promising diagnostic modality.[31] At this time, the precise accuracy of both of these studies has not been determined.

Diagnostic Peritoneal Lavage

Diagnostic peritoneal lavage is quite possibly the greatest step made in diagnosing intra-abdominal trauma in the last 50 years. It has revolutionized the workup of blunt trauma patients. Even with the outstanding accuracy rate found for the technique, it does have its limitations. Peritoneal lavage is of little help in diagnosing retroperitoneal trauma due to the fact that the region is "walled off" from the peritoneal cavity by the posterior peritoneum. As with the other structures of the retroperitoneum, isolated injuries to the diaphragm have not proven to be accurately diagnosed by peritoneal lavage. The false-negative rate has been reported to be 14 to 36% in blunt trauma and 12 to 40% in penetrating trauma.[6,32–34] Occasionally, peritoneal lavage may be helpful when a chest tube has been placed and the lavage fluid is noted to be exiting through the thoracostomy tube, demonstrating a peritoneal-pleural communication.

Pneumoperitoneum

The instillation of 300 to 1000 cc of air into the peritoneal cavity followed by an upright chest radiograph may be diagnostic if the patient develops a pneumothorax. This test must be done in the absence of chest tubes. The procedure is attractive from the standpoint of simplicity and rapidity, but may be associated with air embolism and tension pneumothorax. False-negative tests may occur when the defect is occluded with omentum or intra-abdominal organs. Although some may espouse this technique, the author does not recommend its use due to inaccuracy and danger of complications.

Radioisotopic Studies

Liver scans or liver and spleen scans may be helpful in demonstrating displaced solid organs in the stable patient with suspected diaphragmatic disruption. The most useful view is the right lateral, which shows displacement of the liver superiorly and posteriorly. Kim et al[35] reported excellent results diagnosing right-sided injuries in seven patients. Other authors have proposed the instillation of radioisotopes into either the pleural or peritoneal cavities and scanning for activity in the opposite cavity.[36] The potential exists for false-negative results when the defect is blocked by herniated organs. These studies are also appropriate only in the stable patient.

Thoracoscopy and Laparoscopy

Thoracoscopy and laparoscopy have been proposed as diagnostic techniques that may be helpful in identifying diaphragmatic injuries. Adamthwaite[37] advocates the use of laparoscopy in patients greater than 24 hours after injury and in all patients in the latent phase when all other diagnostic methods have failed to demonstrate a suspected diaphragmatic lesion. Thoracoscopy has been shown to be an effective diagnostic modality when performed in the first 24 hours of injury. After that time, intrapleural adhesions begin to form and the technique becomes technically difficult and the number of inadequate studies increases.[38,39]

The author has found thoracoscopy to be very useful and accurate when used in the stable patient with penetrating trauma to the lower chest. If these patients have no firm indications for exploratory celiotomy, then thoracoscopy, in the author's experience, has been an excellent technique to examine the diaphragm for occult injury. Thoracoscopy is performed in the operating room under general anesthesia using a sterilized pediatric proctoscope introduced though the chest tube insertion site and a probe is inserted anteriorly through a separate stab wound. In this fashion the lung may be manipulated and the entire pleural surface of the diaphragm examined. After the procedure, the chest tube is replaced. If a defect is found in the diaphragm, the patient is prepared for celiotomy and abdominal exploration is performed.

OPERATIVE MANAGEMENT

Acute Phase

The standards of initial trauma resuscitation hold for patients with diaphragmatic injuries. The ABC's of trauma care must be observed and immediate life-threatening injuries attended to. It must be emphasized that pneumatic antishock garments (PASG) are contraindicated in the patient with suspected diaphragmatic disruption. The increase in intra-abdominal pressure may precipitate an acute deterioration in cardiopulmonary status by forcing abdominal viscera up into the thoracic cavity.

In many patients the associated injuries will necessitate exploration and the diaphragmatic injury should be found and surgically addressed at that time. The intra-abdominal and life-threatening injuries should be repaired first and then the diaphragmatic wound should be closed. Rarely, the diaphragmatic injury will take precedence when there is massive disruption and herniation into the thorax or torsion of the heart with compromise of cardiopulmonary function. When this occurs, the herniated viscera should be immediately reduced and the heart placed back into its normal anatomic position.

Some controversy exists over the preferred surgical approach to diagnosed diaphragmatic injuries. Thoracotomy versus celiotomy has been a bone of contention for many years. Most experienced trauma surgeons prefer the abdominal approach for patients in the acute phase. Associated intra-abdominal injuries are present in approximately 85% of patients. These injuries cannot be adequately identified or treated through a thoracotomy. In the series of Waldschmidt and Laws[10] only 1 of 65 patients who initially underwent celiotomy required a subsequent thoracotomy. However, 7 of 15 patients undergoing initial thoracotomy required a celiotomy. The author feels strongly that the only means of addressing the acute diaphragmatic injury is through a midline abdominal incision and exploratory celiotomy.

The midline abdominal incision may also be easily extended into a median sternotomy if the need arises to gain control of the vena cava, improve exposure for hepatic injuries, control mediastinal structures, or insert a vena caval shunt for vascular control of the liver.

The actual closure of the defect may be accomplished in a number of ways and depends to a large extent on the preference and experience of the surgeon. Most surgeons prefer to use a permanent suture rather than absorbable material. Monofilament suture may have a theoretical advantage over braided suture in patients with contamination of the abdominal cavity by spillage of intestinal contents. The technique used to place sutures is highly variable. Some surgeons prefer interrupted horizontal mattress, interrupted figure-of-eight, or interrupted simple sutures, in one or two layers. Other authors have found a running, single layer suture to be adequate.[27] In the acute setting it is, in essence, always possible to close the diaphragmatic defect primarily. Loss of tissue is rarely a factor except in the rare instance of a shotgun wound where tissue loss may be a problem. Synthetic mesh may be necessary in these infrequent cases. The author's preference is for a single layer closure with a permanent monofilament suture, placing overlapping horizontal mattress sutures.

Latent Phase

Concurrent injuries will usually manifest themselves within the first few days post-trauma if operative intervention is required. Therefore the need to explore the abdomen when repairing diaphragmatic injuries months to years after the initial trauma is not a factor. These patients require operative intervention solely to address the diaphragm. The long-standing defect with herniated viscera will often have intrapleural adhesions. For these reasons, it is preferable to approach the chronic diaphragmatic hernia through a thoracotomy. The method of closure remains the same, but the need to resort to synthetic mesh to achieve closure occurs more frequently in the chronic defects. The dissection of adhesions may be tedious and a challenge to the surgeon and if the organs are distended the problems are compounded. Gangrenous viscera may also need to be addressed in the patient presenting with obstruction.

MORBIDITY AND MORTALITY

Acute Phase

The morbidity and mortality in patients with diaphragmatic injuries in the acute phase are dictated by the severity of the associated injuries. Recent series have cited mortality rates of 7 to 28.6%.[16,40–42] All reports related mortality to the associated injuries.

Latent Phase

The rule rather than the exception is for incarceration and strangulation to occur months to years after the traumatic insult. Mortality rates for incarceration have been reported as 20% and for strangulation as 40 to 57%.[43] These figures emphasize the importance of early diagnosis and repair of diaphragmatic injuries to avoid the high mortality rate of late complications.

SUMMARY

Diaphragmatic injuries are a consequence of both blunt and penetrating trauma. The diagnosis of these injuries may be very difficult in the stable patient who does not require exploratory celiotomy for associated injuries. Most disruptions are found at the time of exploration for the associated injuries. The chest radiograph is the most valuable diagnostic tool when it shows an abnormality of one hemidiaphragm. However, the accuracy of the chest radiograph is less than ideal. Diagnostic peritoneal lavage is likewise not very accurate for the diagnosis of isolated diaphragmatic injury. A strong index of suspicion based on the mechanism of injury is probably the most valuable tool in the treatment of the trauma patient with diaphragmatic wounds.

The operative approach to these injuries during the acute phase should be through the abdomen, so that associated injuries may be identified and repaired at the same operation. Likewise, the abdominal exploration should include a painstaking examination of the diaphragm to rule out occult injuries. Chronic diaphragmatic hernias diagnosed during the latent phase should be approached through the chest, since adhesions may be dense and associated intra-abdominal injuries are not a concern.

The high mortality associated with incarcerated and strangulated diaphragmatic hernias emphasize the need for diligent pursuit of a suspected diaphragmatic defect. The natural course of a diaphragmatic injury is to progress to herniation of intra-abdominal contents into the chest cavity. Strangulation, if it occurs, usually presents within 3 years of the traumatic event.

REFERENCES

1. Reid J: Diaphragmatic hernia produced by a penetrating wound. *Edinb Med Surg J* 1840;53:104–107.
2. Paré A: *Oeuvres Completes, vol. 2.* Malgaigne JF (ed). Paris: Bailliere, 1840, pp 94–100.
3. Bowditch HI: Diaphragmatic hernia. *Buffalo Med J* 1853;9:1–39, 65–94.
4. Hedblom CA: Diaphragmatic hernia. *JAMA* 1925;85:947–953.
5. Hood RM: Traumatic diaphragmatic hernia. *Ann Thorac Surg* 1971;12:311–324.
6. Miller OL, Bennett EV, Root HD, et al: Management of penetrating and blunt diaphragmatic injury. *J Trauma* 1984;24:403–409.
7. Robison PD, Harmon PK, Grover FL, et al: The management of penetrating lung injuries in civilian practice. *J Thorac Cardiovasc Surg* 1988;95:184–190.
8. Moore JB, Moore EE, Thompson JS: Abdominal injuries associated with penetrating trauma in the lower chest. *Am J Surg* 1980;140:724–730.
9. Rodkey GV: The management of abdominal injuries. *Surg Clin North Amer* 1966;46:627–644.
10. Waldschmidt ML, Laws HL: Injuries of the diaphragm. *J Trauma* 1980;20:587–592.
11. Drews JA, Mercer EC, Benfield JR: Acute diaphragmatic injuries. *Ann Thorac Surg* 1973;16:67–77.
12. Toh CL, Yeo TT, Chua CL, et al: Diaphragmatic injuries: Why are they overlooked? *J R Coll Surg Edinb* 1991;36:25–28.
13. Agostini E, Sant'Ambrogio G: The diaphragm. In Campbell EJM, Agostini E, Davie JN (eds): *The Respiratory Muscles: Mechanics and Neural Control*, 2nd ed. Philadelphia: WB Saunders, 1970, pp 145–160.
14. Hill LD: Injuries of the diaphragm following blunt trauma. *Surg Clin North Am* 1972;52:611–624.
15. Patten BM: *Foundations of Embryology*, 2nd ed. New York: McGraw-Hill Book Co, 1964.
16. Sharma OP: Traumatic diaphragmatic rupture: Not an uncommon entity—personal experience with a collective review of the 1980s. *J Trauma* 1989;29:678–682.
17. Jarrett F, Bernhardt LC: Right-sided diaphragmatic injury: Rarity or overlooked diagnosis. *Arch Surg* 1978;113:737–739.
18. Hardy JJ: Closed traumatic rupture of the diaphragm. *Aust NZ J Surg* 1966;35:222–225.
19. van Loenhout RMM, Schiphorst TJMJ, Wittens CHA, et al: Traumatic intrapericardial diaphragmatic hernia. *J Trauma* 1986;26:271–275.
20. Brooks VS: Intrapericardial diaphragmatic hernia. *Br J Surg* 1952;40:511–513.
21. Bernatz PE, Burnside AF Jr, Clagett OT: Problem of the ruptured diaphragm. *JAMA* 1958;168:877–881.
22. Marchand P: A study of the forces productive of gastro-oesophageal regurgitation and herniation through the diaphragmatic hiatus. *Thorax* 1957;12:189–194.
23. Comroe JH: *Physiology of Respiration*, 2nd ed. Chicago: Year Book Medical Publisher, 1974, p 98.
24. Ebert PA, Gaertner RA, Zuidema GD: Traumatic diaphragmatic hernia. *Surg Gynecol Obstet* 1967;125:59–65.
25. Sullivan RE: Strangulation and obstruction in diaphragmatic hernia due to direct trauma. Report of two cases and review of the English literature. *J Thorac Cardiovasc Surg* 1966;52:725–734.
26. Negre J, Teerenhovi O, Autio V: Hepatic coma resulting from diaphragmatic rupture and hepatic herniation. *Arch Surg* 1986;121:950–951.
27. Laws HL, Hawkins ML: Diaphragmatic injury. *Adv Trauma* 1987;2:207–228.
28. Carter BN, Giuseff J: Strangulated diaphragmatic hernia. *Ann Surg* 1948;128:210–225.
29. Wise L, Connor J, Hwang YH, et al: Traumatic injuries to the diaphragm. *J Trauma* 1973;13:946–950.
30. Johnson CD: Blunt injuries of the diaphragm. *Br J Surg* 1988;75:226–230.
31. Mirvis SE, Keramati B, Buckman R, et al: MR imaging of traumatic diaphragmatic rupture. *J Comp Assist Tomo* 1988;12:147–149.
32. Freeman T, Fischer RP: The inadequacy of peritoneal lavage in diagnosing acute diaphragmatic rupture. *J Trauma* 1976;16:538–542.
33. Aronoff RJ, Reynolds J, Thal ER: Evaluation of diaphragmatic injuries. *Am J Surg* 1982;144:671–674.
34. Thal ER: Evaluation of peritoneal lavage and local exploration of lower chest and abdominal stab wounds. *J Trauma* 1977;17:642–648.
35. Kim EE, McConnell BJ, McConnell RW, et al: Radionuclide diagnosis of diaphragmatic rupture with herniation. *Surgery* 1983;94:36–40.
36. Pecoraro JP, Shea LM, Tenorio LE, et al: Radioisotope-assisted diagnosis of traumatic rupture of the diaphragm. *Am Surg* 1985;51:687–689.
37. Adamthwaite DN: Traumatic diaphragmatic hernia: A new indication for laparoscopy. *Br J Surg* 1984;71:315.
38. Jackson AM, Ferreira AA: Thoracoscopy as an aid to diagnosis of diaphragmatic injury in penetrating wounds of the left lower chest. *Injury* 1976;7:213–217.
39. Adamthwaite DN: Penetrating injury of the diaphragm. *Injury* 1982;14:151–158.

40. Rodriquez-Morales G, Rodriguez A, Shatney CH: Acute rupture of the diaphragm in blunt trauma: Analysis of 60 patients. *J Trauma* 1986;26:438–444.
41. van Vugt AB, Schoots FJ: Acute diaphragmatic rupture due to blunt trauma: A retrospective analysis. *J Trauma* 1989;29:683–686.
42. Voeller GR, Reisser JR, Fabian TC, et al: Blunt diaphragm injuries: A five-year experience. *Am Surg* 1990;56:28–31.
43. Harman PK, Root HD: Injury to the diaphragm. In Mattox KL, Moore EE, Feliciano DV (eds): *Trauma*. Norwalk, CT: Appleton and Lange, 1988, p 426.

Index